T0353776

THE PRECIOUS SECRETS OF THE FOETAL CIRCULATION

The 8th Centenary Edition

Alan Gilchrist

AuthorHouse™ UK
1663 Liberty Drive
Bloomington, IN 47403 USA
www.authorhouse.co.uk
UK TFN: 0800 0148641 (Toll Free inside the UK)
UK Local: 02036 956322 (+44 20 3695 6322 from outside the UK)

Because of the dynamic nature of the Internet, any web addresses or links contained in this book may have changed
since publication and may no longer be valid. The views expressed in this work are solely those of the author and do
not necessarily reflect the views of the publisher, and the publisher hereby disclaims any responsibility for them.

Any people depicted in stock imagery provided by Getty Images are models,
and such images are being used for illustrative purposes only.
Certain stock imagery © Getty Images.

This book is printed on acid-free paper.

ISBN: 979-8-8230-8966-1 (sc)
ISBN: 979-8-8230-8967-8 (e)

Library of Congress Control Number: 2024918648

Print information available on the last page.

Published by AuthorHouse 01/14/2025

authorHOUSE®

Dedication

'From the generosity of my parents, James and Ivy Gilchrist, and the bravery of my brothers, Jim and Neil, I was able to become a doctor and work in Africa, where I married Pauline. To all five this book is dedicated'.

About the Front Cover Illustration

The front cover, it represents Aesculapius, the Greek god of medicine, trying to understand what happens in the mother when she is pregnant. When I was in Zimbabwe, I asked my gardener to sit on the other side of my desk holding a stick which had been left behind by a patient of mine after an operation, and I sketched him.

Acknowledgements

To my son Andrew and his wife Kim, who live in Oswestry, I thank them for many years of comfort they gave me after returning to England in 2013. To Graham Jones, a sheep farmer near Oswestry, who gave me several stillborn lambs, I am grateful. These were of vital importance to the confirmation of the similarity between the circulation in the human foetus, and that of the sheep foetus, both of which I had discovered in Africa. I am also grateful to Kevin Battams of Battams Butchery Oswestry, for providing me with parts of a lamb's anatomy, as I had asked. These allowed me to see the difference between the lamb's anatomy and that of the foetus, and to suggest what may happen at birth. I thank my friend John Quinn, a professional photographer, who came out of retirement and helped me with my book in many ways. Another friend who deserves my thanks is Ben Hillidge, an IT specialist whose contribution complimented John's. After my stroke in June 2022, my daughter Mary Kirkman, invited me to stay with her and her husband Bernard and family in Horley. It was a happy move. Mary has helped a lot with the secretarial work. After several years of divorce from AuthorHouse UK, we are now happily reunited, with the outcome you may see in the following pages. I must not forget to thank the DWP for the generous financial support it has given me ever since I returned from Africa in 2013.

My story begins in a biology class when I was a medical student, and I heard about two streams of blood, one venous and the other arterial in the same chamber of a foetal heart. I wondered how it was done. Somewhere in the deep recesses of my memory, I kept that problem locked away from consciousness and it resurfaced many years later when I was working in Africa. I will tell you of the many things that happened in the intervening years, because they may have been links in the long chain which had led up to the eruption of my buried thoughts.

In the warm summer of 1947, I was a student in the Central Middlesex Hospital in west London, which was a sector of The Middlesex Hospital in the centre of London. I was athletics captain, and during training had developed a painful foot. I was referred for physiotherapy and fell in love most strongly with the young lady who massaged my foot. My love for her so affected me that I could not concentrate on my studies. I was supposed to be studying pathology, and my performance in the final exams was poor. I had won a prize as the most promising student in the first year, but I knew I had just scraped through when I qualified in November 1949. In 1947, my father became 65 and retired from his work in London. In 1930 he had built a holiday bungalow near the north Kent coast, and on retirement my parents settled there. I had to move into digs and missed the comfort and companionship of home during those difficult years.

In those days, we could go straight into medical practice after qualifying; but most did not do this, we lined up for interviews with the eminent consultants to compete for their prestigious house appointments. I did not want to stay at The Middlesex, I had had enough of studying. I was worried that I would not be able to cope with an accident. We had had a talk by a surgeon from the Birmingham Accident Hospital, and I was anxious to go there. I did go to Birmingham and worked as a house surgeon in the casualty department for six months. It was a dream come true, I was involved in every kind of accident and learned ten times more in those six months than my colleagues back home.

The six consultant surgeons were all British, but we, the registrars, housemen, and anaesthetists, were a motley crew. Some were Czechs and Poles from the tired post-war heart of Eastern Europe, and there were a few Irish doctors as well. We began to see patients from overseas, including the Caribbean. I was in a new environment, a different city from my own London. Different people, different accents, and a different surrounding countryside. It was all something extra, a bonus for not wanting a job at the Middlesex. But also, there was something very special that I was to see, which I would have missed in London. At Christmas time the nurses were to have an outing to the Shakespeare Memorial Theatre in Stratford on Avon. The casualty sister invited me to join them. We were taken by coach to see 'Toad of Toad Hall,' an adaptation by A.A. Milne of Kenneth Grahame's 'The Wind in the Willows,' my favourite book, which my father had given me at Christmas when I was ten. It was the finest piece of theatre I had seen, only equalled by 'The Mikado' at Sadler's Wells, when our family went to see it in the summer holidays just before the war.

I was never very good at waking and getting out of bed quickly. When I was in digs in London with a fellow student, our landlady, Mrs. Hewitt, a Geordie, used to say I wasn't asleep, I was unconscious. Later, in Birmingham, when I was supposed to be in theatre, I was sound asleep in bed. The door was thrown open roughly. 'Gilchrist' shouted the surgeon, half-dressed ready to operate, without knocking or waiting to be invited in. I sheepishly got dressed and went to the theatre without breakfast or anything to say, with my head held low as I held retractors for him. But I did well in that job, and towards the end of my six months he would have liked me to stay on.

Our registrar taught me how to suture properly, and how to do the 'Gillies' stich, introduced by Sir Harold Gillies, a famous New Zealand plastic surgeon. One of the most important things I learned in Birmingham was the importance of doing hospital internships before being let loose on the unsuspecting public. Some years later, newly qualified doctors had to do house jobs before being registered with the General Medical Council as a qualified doctor and allowed to practise and seek further employment elsewhere. More importantly, Birmingham had given me a coat of armour, which allowed me to wade into an accident with confidence. I could never forget Birmingham, my very first job, and all the valuable things I learned there.

Then came National Service. Both my elder and younger brothers had volunteered for military service during the war when they were underage. I did not do this, and in October 1943 I went straight from school to medical school. Those who had missed war service had to do two years national service and three summer camps after the war, and after my stay in Birmingham I was glad to be called up on 9th July 1950. During our initial training, which included military drill, we were asked where we would want to serve, and I chose Malaya. After five weeks I was posted to Donnington in Shropshire, and a month later was allowed to go home for a weekend to see my parents before boarding a troopship at Southampton. My mother was seriously ill with a widespread rash and a chest infection.

When my younger brother was sixteen, he asked our doctor to pass him fit for military service, but the doctor refused. When he turned seventeen, he went to the doctor again, and the doctor gave in and allowed him to join up. During training in the winter of 1943-4, he developed pneumonia and died in Chester Military Hospital on Easter Day, 2nd April 1944. When I kissed his head as he lay dying, I smelt a strange smell in his breath. I did not know what it was; in my own mind I called it the smell of death, and as I bent down and kissed my mother goodbye, I smelt the same smell and knew she was dying. (I have recently understood that the smell would have been that of acetone, one of the three ketone bodies which occur in ketosis shortly before death).

My brain was in a turmoil as I travelled that evening to our depot. The next morning, instead of catching the boat train for Southampton, I went to the War Office in London and met the senior medical officials on the top floor. They allowed me to take my mother to hospital, and we travelled together by ambulance to the Middlesex, where a clever medical registrar diagnosed Systemic Lupus Erythematosus, (S.L.E), and put her on mepacrine, one of the newer antimalarials which made her yellow. She very gradually improved, and after many weeks was allowed to return home. Meanwhile, I was posted to Eastern Command and worked throughout the winter in one of the wards in Colchester Military Hospital. I became very depressed there and asked the major in charge if I could have a week's holiday. He referred me to a young army psychiatrist who said I had had a breakdown and downgraded me to 'Base only.' In the spring my mother had regained much of her strength, and I wrote to the War Office and asked if I could be sent to Malaya. I was referred to the senior medical colonel in Eastern Command, who shouted at me 'You can't write to the War Office. Get out, you're on the next boat,' I was happy again.

(Years later, I understood how my mother had developed that dreadful condition of S.L.E. My father owned a half-acre plot opposite our bungalow. It had a simple wire fence which separated it from nearby farmland. He burnt rubbish on the plot, and in the height of hot midsummer 1950, the fire which he had lit, spread outside the plot near to a field of wheat ready to be gathered. My father and mother battled desperately to save the wheat, in the heat of the sun above and the heat of the fire below. They almost lost the battle and became completely exhausted as they managed to put out the fire inches away from the wheat. My mother's illness began shortly afterwards. It is an autoimmune disease, much more common in women, with sunlight being a common causal factor, and with a high mortality rate. My father would have been 68, and my mother 10 years younger. In 1965 when my father died, my mother went to live in New Zealand close to her daughter and family. She continued to lead an active life, looking after herself in her flat, up to a few days before her death in March 1981, 30 years after her illness, when she was 88.)

In a week I was on the Empire Trooper, an old German ship taken by Britain after the war. We chugged away from Southampton at a steady 13 knots. I was the only doctor travelling out east, and shared a cabin with an officer in the Pay Corps. He strongly impressed on me that I was first an officer and then a gentleman, not the other way round. But later, I heard he fiddled the books and was arrested and became neither the one nor the other. The ship's medical officer was a major, having volunteered for four year's national service. Below decks were several hundred troops. Our first port of call was Gibraltar, and we went ashore and stretched our legs up the main street. The cobwebs had mainly blown away and I was feeling a new man. We next reached Port Said and passed through the Suez Canal into the Red Sea. We were on a luxury cruise taking us halfway round the world, with nothing to do but lounge on deck and watch the flying fish and porpoises alongside. I had three good meals a day served by waiters from Goa, and two pips on each shoulder. I was beginning to enjoy army life.

Later, we reached Aden on the southern tip of the Arabian Peninsula at midnight and stopped for fuel. When we reached the Indian ocean, the major asked me to give the troops some instruction on first aid. There were six national service dentists travelling with us, and the major arranged for them to teach us two some dentistry, in the middle of the Indian Ocean. I remember teeth are not pulled out; they are pushed out!

We stopped at Colombo in beautiful Ceylon, then departed for Singapore. Being downgraded to base only, I did not go up north, but stayed in Singapore and worked in the newly built Gurkha hospital. The Gurkhas were fine, brave, and well-disciplined soldiers, each carrying a terrible curved kukri knife. There was a close bond between them and their British counterparts. In the hospital clinic I met many of them. They came from the high isolated valleys in mountainous Nepal, each with part of his name reflecting his valley of origin. I also saw a few of the British Gurkhas. I shook hands with one of them and he could not open his hand easily; he had the rare condition of Myotonia Congenita where muscles fail to relax after contraction. It is associated with premature baldness, which was easily seen when he removed his hat. He was embarrassed when I told him about his condition; he had served the army well without the authorities knowing about it and wished to keep it that way. I understood this and we said no more about it. I had my own secret disability and knew how he felt. On 9th July 1951 I received another pip on each shoulder and became a captain. It was part of national service routine for medical officers in the R.A.M.C. (Royal Army Medical Corps), who had served for a year. I picked up a bit of Gurkhali in Singapore; 'deri ramro bundabust,' a very good arrangement. When I went to the bank in Singapore, it was like walking into a fridge. It was the first time I had been in such a modern ventilated building.

After five months in Singapore, I was posted up country to Headquarters Malaya in Kuala Lumpur (KL). There were two medical posts there, one for the troops and the other for the families. But due to a shortage of medical officers they were combined, and I took over both. I ran the sick parades for the troops in the mornings and visited the families in the afternoons. They gave me a car and taught me to drive. For me it was a new way of running things, with wives and children in KL somewhere behind the front line.

My father forwarded a questionnaire from the British Medical Association, asking for details of my health and smoking habits. They were investigating the connection between smoking and lung cancer. Five years later they followed up with another, the results of which established smoking as the cause. Two thirds of smoking doctors had dropped the habit and the rate of heart attacks in doctors began to fall. There was also a link between smoking and many other health problems. Smoking had increased in women, and by 1986 lung cancer caught up with breast cancer as the leading cause of death in women. Smoking became associated with unsuccessful pregnancies, intrauterine growth retardation and increased infant mortality, and there was an increased risk of respiratory infections in children which could leave them with residual lung damage, caused by smoking in mothers, which became known as passive smoking. In 1983 the Royal College of Physicians issued a warning; of every thousand young men who smoked, one would be murdered, six would die on the roads, but 250 would die prematurely from tobacco-related health conditions. The WHO called smoking the biggest preventable health hazard to mankind. The BMA study and other similar pioneer studies resulted in the slow but sure reduction in the widespread smoking habit, which had caused countless deaths. (The information given here is accurate, I have extracted it from something I had written earlier, which was my answer to a question in the entrance exam for the College of Primary Care Physicians of Zimbabwe. I had spent several evenings working late in our medical school library, poring over old dusty medical journals).

In 1945, the Middlesex Hospital celebrated its second centenary, and on one weekend opened every part of the hospital and medical school to the public. Jack Howell, a fellow student, who later became president of the BMA and professor of medicine at the Southampton School of Medicine, asked me to help with a demonstration for the visitors in the physiology lab. He sat me in front of the visitors and asked me to hyperventilate, (breathe deeply and fast). I did it as hard as I could and began to feel strange sensations throughout my body, like electric currents. Then my muscles began to contract, with my fingers pressing against my thumbs, and my hands and feet flexing. My knees and elbows became flexed, my lips were pursed together, and my eyes were tightly closed. I had sort of paralysed myself, (except for my respiratory muscles). After about twelve minutes Jack called a halt. He thought I had acted well, but it was all genuine. It taught me a lot, and I met many cases of hyperventilation later in my medical career. In KL, I saw some cases in the troops, the first being in the hot kitchen with the cook having flexed fingers. One day I was driving past a game of soccer and saw the goalie get the ball kicked hard into his stomach. He collapsed onto the ground. I stopped and went over to him. His fingers were tightly pressed together. He recovered. A soldier in pain arrived at the medical centre on a stretcher. He had an acute appendix, and his fingers were tightly flexed. The climate in Malaya was very hot and humid, and we all sweated a lot. I think it had been difficult for some Europeans to adjust to the new environment, and they may have copied the dogs subconsciously by keeping cool by panting.

We may have had a few cases of malaria, probably benign tertian, because I became interested in the spleen, especially percussion of it. I found that the lower limit of normal splenic dullness was 4 of my fingerbreadths above the left costal margin. I could detect an enlargement of the spleen when the dullness was 3 fingerbreadths above the costal margin, before the spleen was palpable on deep inspiration, and on one occasion the dullness was higher than normal, 5 fingerbreadths above. In chronic malaria the spleen may be larger than normal, but in this case, I assumed it had shrunk from fibrosis. See diagram D 1.

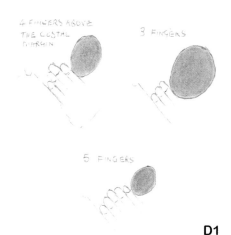

D1

We had some excellent men in Malaya. General Gerald Templer arrived when I was there, and soon the Emergency began to come to an end. Colonel Alec Drummond, Director of the Army Medical Services in Malaya, was a live wire who was always on the go and kept in touch with all the medical units there. He often popped into the Medical Centre where I worked. We had a good crew in the Centre, headed by Sgt. Smith, a Scot. There was also a cheerful chubby nursing sister, also from Scotland, who taught me how to pierce ears, and we had two young National Service orderlies from England.

Colonel Drummond later became Sir Alec Drummond, Director General of the Royal Army Medical Corps. He was very friendly towards me, and once invited me to afternoon tea with his wife when he was going up country. She was young and attractive, and I wasn't at ease, but she had another lady with her which helped to loosen my tongue.

In the officer's mess, I sat with men and a few ladies of various branches of the military, including the army pilots who flew the light Auster spotter planes, an occasional Aussie, and the National Service dentist Freddie Townsend. I palled up with Fred and a young chap in the R.A.F., Don Webb. Sometimes, in the cooler evenings, we three would go down to the Selangor golf club in my car for a drink. Every Sunday lunch was a delicious Indian curry, prepared by our expert Indian chefs. After lunch we three would monopolise the snooker table, where they taught me about gamesmanship. Don had to attend an H.Q. meeting and told me how a British colonel had nothing to say except 'We need more wire,' and 'The National Servicemen are absolutely first class.'

After seven months in Kuala Lumpur, my National Service was coming to an end, and I prepared for the journey back home. On the day I left KL, Alec Drummond came to say goodbye, and said I did a bloody good job, as we shook hands. At Singapore I boarded the Empire Pride, and we sped home much faster than the old Empire Trooper. I picked up a little Malay in KL. A pretty eight- year- old daughter of a Eurasian officer made it up herself and taught it to me, with a twinkle in her eye. She had probably heard the original from her father. 'Satu ampat jalan.' 1, 4, the road.

I loved Malaya, its colour and warmth, and its multicultural population. It was prosperous, producing half the world's rubber and half the world's tin, I was told. Because of the year there I regained a lot of my self-respect and self-confidence which had left me in those two difficult years as a student, compounded by my downgrading. I was determined to make up for the ground I had lost and decided on a career in surgery. In the middle of the Indian ocean, this time going home, I worked out my plans. First, I would do a year's pathology, then house jobs in medicine and surgery before attempting to climb the surgical ladder. During my two years' National Service, I had picked up a fair amount of clinical acumen, and there was more to come, much more.

I was de-mobbed on 9th July 1952, and after a month in the laboratory of the Royal Free Hospital where I learned about the maturation of the red cells, I went up to the General Hospital Nottingham as a Senior House Officer, (S.H.O), Pathology, for a year. Nottingham was all that I would have wished for. If Birmingham was King of the Midlands, Nottingham was its Queen. The people were proud of their city, you could sense it. My year there proved to be an enlightening experience. The year's work was divided into quarters, haematology, bacteriology, biochemistry, and morbid histology. The day usually started with a short walk from the lab to the mortuary, where I attended the post-mortems. On the wall outside the mortuary was a plaque which indicated where King Charles 1st had raised his standard in 1642. It would have been exactly where the post-mortems were performed, and three hundred and ten years later, I was raising *my standard of medicine* on the same spot. Eventually, I performed many of the post-mortems myself and wrote detailed notes on them. I still have my book containing the notes. Although the post-mortems were important and carried out carefully by the pathologist and me, we were not involved with the forensic cases. They were performed by the Director of the lab who was a forensic pathologist who attended court to give expert evidence which could affect the lives of the defendants.

I slotted in with the lab technicians and helped with the routine work. I was learning about all the tests a laboratory would be asked to do and performing them myself. In the evenings and at weekends, I was on call for all the emergency work, and in charge of the large blood bank which served the hospital and the whole of the County of Nottingham and beyond.

Early in 1953, the Royal College of Surgeons announced they were creating a new degree for anaesthetists and were to hold a week's course in pharmacology and anaesthetics at the College in London. I was allowed to go on the course, which would help me pass future surgical examinations. Next door to the lecture hall was the famous John Hunter Museum. Each lunch hour and in the evenings after the lectures, I examined all the specimens systematically. At the back of the museum was a perspex case containing two spleens from cases of chronic malaria, one larger and the other smaller than normal, which confirmed my finding in Kuala Lumpur of a small spleen in chronic malaria. The visit to the College was turning out to be more than a course of lectures, and there were still other interesting specimens to come, lying in wait for me at the front of the museum. I came across them on my last day at the College, two beautiful casts of the lungs. The bronchi and pulmonary vessels had been injected with resin and painted in different colours, while the other tissues had been removed with acid. I noticed a pattern in the relationship of the bronchi and vessels, but there was no description of it nearby, and for those interested in the anatomy of the lung, this is the pattern I noticed.

If you take a key ring and hold it out horizontally, then you can pull out a key on each side horizontally. Imagine the keys to be the bronchi painted green, with the pulmonary arteries in blue lying above them, and the pulmonary veins in red lying below. Now, without twisting the keys you can find the relationship of the bronchi and vessels in any part of the lungs. For example, with the right lung, swing the right key up vertically. The pulmonary artery will lie medial to the bronchus and the pulmonary vein laterally.

Swing it down vertically through 180 degrees, and the artery will be lateral and the vein medial. Swing it round to the front of the ring, the artery will in front of the bronchus, with the vein behind. Swing it up through 180 degrees, the artery will lie behind and the vein in front. Swing it round to the back of the ring, the artery will be in front, with the vein behind. Swing it down through 180 degrees, the artery will be behind and the vein in front. These manoeuvres can be repeated on the left side to give a mirror image of the positions in the right lung. The exercise could be repeated using a small fan, with the unexpanded blades held horizontally, and with blue paint on top and red paint below on each blade. Open the fan into three quarters of a circle and swivel it round forwards and backwards with the same result as with the keys. I noticed that the arteries followed this pattern fairly faithfully, but the relationship of the veins to the bronchi was not so constant. In the upper lobes the bronchi and vessels were crowded together, but in the lower lobes there was more space between them. In the upper lobes the arteries would lie central to the bronchi, with the veins lying peripherally. In the lower lobes the arteries would lie outside the bronchi and the veins inside, with a gradual change in the position from above downwards. Diagram D 2.

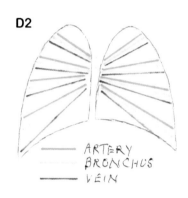

I returned to Nottingham and continued my work there. After three months' haematology I went to bacteriology, where the senior technician showed me how to examine urines properly. This was one of the most important things I learned there. I became interested in the examination of the cerebrospinal fluid, (c.s.f.), especially in cases of tuberculous meningitis. In the mortuary I had seen cases, with a thick green exudate on the lower surface of the brain. In contrast, it was unusual to find tubercule bacilli in the c.s.f., which the clinicians sent us after lumbar puncture. Why should the organisms cause so much mischief and almost disappear without trace? It was an enigma, a paradox. Even in those days, T.B. was a scourge and difficult to treat, though streptomycin had become an important drug in its treatment. The bacillus was discovered by Robert Koch, a G.P., in his home in 1882. I remember the date well; it was the same as my father's birthday. The lab routine for examining the c.s.f., for T.B., was first to examine the fluid in the bottle with a watchmaker's eyeglass to see if it was clear and colourless. It may have been reported clear, but I found it was only clear if it contained less than 40 cells per cu mm. Next, we checked the protein, sugar, and chlorides, did the cell count and culture, centrifuged and examined the deposit after staining with the Ziehl-Neelsen stain and washing with acid and alcohol. This stained the leucocytes blue and the T.B. pink. As I have said, it was unusual to find the bacilli. This was a challenge for me, and I decided to make a special effort to find them. First, I centrifuged well and made sure there was a tightly packed deposit at the bottom of the centrifuge tube. Then I poured all the deposit carefully onto a glass slide in a long thin narrow strip, and after drying, fixed and stained it. I then put the slide in my drawer and went down to supper. After supper I returned to the lab and examined the slide systematically with the oil-immersion lens, not missing a cell. The strips were only a few cells wide, and when I came to the end of a row, I moved the strip to the next row and examined every cell in the opposite direction. Time went by without finding T.B. One hour passed, then another half hour, then after nearly two hours I saw three pink bacilli peeping out from under the edge of one of the blue leucocytes. I took the Vernier reading on my microscope stage, finished the rest of the slide without finding any more and put the slide in my drawer. The next morning, I checked the Vernier, saw the bacilli again and showed them to the senior technician. A report went out that morning to the physicians who had already made the diagnosis and started treatment. Acid and alcohol fast bacilli present. I found the tubercule bacilli twice more in the bacteriology lab, before moving to the next section. The only way to find T.B. in the c.s.f., is to examine every cell of the centrifuged deposit.

I learned so much in Nottingham, which was precious for me and occupies a central place in my medical memories. Pathology, so important, I am glad I went to Nottingham, it laid my future medical career on a solid firm basis and helped me through each part.

During my stay in Nottingham, I was called to be medically re-examined by a senior army psychiatrist who strongly denied that I had had a breakdown and upgraded me.

After Nottingham I went up to the cold cut-off corner of north-eastern England in the autumn of 1953, and became a house physician in the Darlington Memorial Hospital, treating live patients again. I became involved with a wealth of clinical material there, and I cannot speak too highly of the way it was managed by the three physicians, and how well the patients were treated by the nursing staff. There were lots of minor procedures to do, putting up drips, paracentesis abdominis and lumbar punctures. I often had to inject streptomycin intrathecally into a little girl with T.B. meningitis. In those days we did not have dipsticks and examined urines for sugar and protein the old-fashioned way in the sluice room. The most common condition I met there was chronic bronchitis with right heart failure. Some men may have been gassed in the Great War; others had been miners. The diuretic we used was mersalyl. Wherever I went for my hospital jobs I played tennis, if I could find a partner. In Nottingham I had to sweep the rain off the court before we could play, in Darlington it was the snow. One of the G.P.'s held a party at Christmas. When I met his wife, she said 'He's just a student.' I took it as a compliment, perhaps my epitaph. I have a soft spot for Darlington now, but I did not appreciate having to get up in those chilly nights that that part of the country seemed to specialise in.

So, I was glad to find another house job in Canterbury where it was warmer, and I was there from spring until autumn in 1954. The job was part general surgery and part genito-urinary. Neither of the two registrars who were from overseas were very generous. They wanted to do as much operating as they could, and the housemen picked up the crumbs. But I learned a lot there, just holding retractors, how to repair an inguinal hernia, how to resect bowel and do the anastomosis, how to do a prostatectomy and how to catheterise. I often had to get up at night to relieve the clot retention that might follow a prostatectomy. I suppose much of the work was a repetition of what we had been taught, or should have been taught, in our clinical years at medical school, but the housemen were more closely involved day and night. In Darlington, the houseman was really the central figure in the play, but in Canterbury, though I may have worked long hours without a break, I was relegated to playing a minor role. 'House Surgeon' was really an inappropriate title.

In the early 1950's, when I did my four hospital internships, the junior doctors were on duty 24 hours a day. Years later, sessions were introduced which limited the daily number of hours to be worked by the junior doctors.

Towards the end of my stay in Canterbury I was stopped in the corridor by one of the pathologists. He knew I had done the path job in Nottingham. His pathologist friend in Bulawayo, Southern Rhodesia, wanted an assistant. Would I be interested? I was curious. I eventually accepted. It took me to Africa.

Southern Rhodesia, now the independent country of Zimbabwe, was part of the Central African Federation of Rhodesia and Nyasaland, which had been created in 1953 by joining prosperous Northern and Southern Rhodesia to poorer Nyasaland with few natural resources. Northern Rhodesia is now the independent country of Zambia and Nyasaland is now Malawi.

I arrived in Bulawayo in December 1954 when I was 30. The pathologist had booked me into a hotel in the suburbs of Bulawayo, which had a three-storey block of rooms. My room was on the ground floor, and I was bothered by mosquitoes. After some months I was moved to the first floor, where there were fewer mosquitoes, and eventually I was on the top floor and virtually mosquito-free. My first lesson on malaria management, which shows how the rural African, living at ground level is disadvantaged.

The dining room was in the main house, and I shared the table with other immigrants who had recently arrived in the Federation. I palled up with a young South African, and we played tennis together. He invited me to join him in the local Multi-racial Society. The meetings were held monthly. Apparently, two Africans had been elected to each of the three Federal territories. One of them for Southern Rhodesia was Mr. Hove, a local Bulawayo man, who attended the meetings frequently. I believe that when the Federation began, a gradual increase in African participation in the running of the country was part of the Constitution.

The path. job did not work out; from the start we did not get on well together. I had had a very good reference from Nottingham, which had been seen by the Middlesex medical consultant son in law of my new boss, and which had led to my being accepted. No cheery greeting as I stepped off the plane in Bulawayo, no friendly moments in the lab. For the first time since qualifying, I had had a setback. All three consultants in Darlington had given me very good and encouraging references, and the surgeon in Birmingham had wanted me to stay. Of course, my new boss had been brave opening a new laboratory in Bulawayo, he was a pioneer. What he needed was financial help to carry him through the difficult early days of the only private laboratory in Bulawayo, and I was no good for him.

My work was mainly routine haematology, with blood counts and differential counts, which was easier than at Nottingham, where I had begun to examine bone marrows, and where I had been competent enough with blood grouping and cross-matching to run the blood bank. However, the hours were good, and the pay more than a houseman's. I bought a car and explored the environs of Bulawayo. I visited Cecil Rhodes' grave in the Matopos hills thirty miles away and played tennis on the sand courts around Bulawayo. I joined a tennis club and played further away, in the farming and mining areas. My year's contract was not renewed, and at the end of 1955 I did not return home. I wanted to see Lake Nyasa and work with the African people up north. I drove up to Salisbury the capital, now called Harare, and met Richard Morris, the first Federal Secretary for Health. I said if he would send me up to Nyasaland, I would join the government medical service. He offered me Fort Johnston at the south end of the lake, and I gladly accepted. With him at that meeting was Dyson Blair, his deputy, and another doctor who gave me some advice on what to carry to Fort Johnston; nothing posh, just a few knives and forks from Woolworth's etc. and a light mac. Richard Morris had arranged a party that evening for the Federal ministers, and he invited me to join them. Having come with my sports jacket, I was conspicuous as the only one without a suit. I met his wife and daughter, and all the ministers; they were a fine group of well-built healthy-looking men. I mentioned to Richard Morris that I had planned to drive down to Cape Town before starting my work up north, and he recommended a good hotel where I could stay.

I was soon on my way in my Morris minor station wagon, doing about 50 miles an hour, and being overtaken all the time by large fast American cars. The hotel in Cape Town was as good as recommended, and I spent a comfortable week there exploring the city. It had a reputation as being very windy, with all the four seasons in the same day. My next stop was Grahamstown, and I arrived there late on Christmas Eve, where the hotel evening meal had finished, and the dining room closed. I got up early before breakfast on Christmas Day and headed for the Transkei, feeling quite peckish without a good meal since Cape Town. I arrived at Umtata, the capital of the province that evening, and the owner of the Grosvener hotel invited me to join him and his family for the Christmas supper. I departed the next morning in good humour and headed along the Garden Route for warm Durban on the coast. I spent a couple of easy days in Durban, then headed for the long road to Johannesburg, and I arrived there in the early afternoon. Now when I was four, a business friend of my father came to say goodbye to us, before leaving for South Africa. I remember the occasion well because he shook my hand so tightly. He had become very successful in his work and was now a senior man in a biscuit factory in Johannesburg. I wanted to meet him again and stopped my car in the middle of Joburg. On the other side of the road a man came out of the building opposite. I went over and asked if he knew where the Premier biscuit factory was. He replied, why do you want to know, and I said I want to meet Mr.J.F., and he said I had lunch with him today. Now, even in those days Joburg was a big city and it was such an incredible coincidence to meet him. He led me to J.F.'s house, and I walked up the front path and knocked on the door. J.F. opened the door and I gave him a firm handshake. Such a happy meeting, he brought me in, and I met his wife and two children. The next day, his wife took me round Joburg, to see the Zoo Park and other places too.

After two days I left and headed northwards, re-entering Southern Rhodesia, and stopping in Bulawayo to pick up my belongings. I then headed northwest and crossed the Zambezi at the Victoria Falls. 'Mosi owa tunya', the smoke that thunders, such a grand picture, the best natural geographical feature I had ever seen. I continued my way through Northern Rhodesia to Lusaka, then headed east towards the border with Nyasaland. The wide all-weather dirt roads were well-kept by graders going each way, as I passed them. Near the Nyasaland border was a large seminary. I stopped and met the mother superior, who asked me to kneel and pray with her. Such a refreshing moment in my long and dusty journey without a companion. My memories of those days are not always clear. All I can say is that I entered the Nyasaland border somewhere and drove down to Salisbury, recrossing the Zambezi at Tete and booking into a Salisbury hotel. On 1st January 1956, which was a Sunday, I booked into the Salisbury hospital, causing a commotion, because nobody expected me to arrive before the Monday. Eventually, the medical superintendent appeared, and we had a little chat and arranged for me to start work the next day.

After several weeks training I was posted to Mtoko, to relieve the doctor there who was ill, and after another two weeks I was on my way up north to Fort Johnston. The road led to the Zambezi, which we crossed in a large barge carrying several cars, pulled by another vessel, at Tete in Portuguese East Africa. The next part could hardly be called a road, it was more like a dried-up rocky riverbed, surrounded by bush or nothing. Further on, I was involved in a ridiculous incident. An old large American car, packed with people, crested the hill a hundred yards in front of me, in a cloud of dust and came to a halt with his front bumper resting on mine. 'We keep to the left in this country', he waved to me. I did not move, and pointed to the side where there was room to pass. He took off his brake and started to push my little car backwards. I reversed and drove off on the left, fuming inside, and arrived in Fort Johnston safely in a better temper.

Fort Johnston.

Fort Johnston, now renamed Mangoche, was a small township on the west side of the river Shire, pronounced like She-eerie, five miles south of the bar, where the river flowed southwards from Lake Nyasa and joined the Zambezi. The 'Calendar Lake' as it was called by some, was magnificent and beautiful, 365 miles long and 52 miles wide at its widest point. The water was fresh and potable with an abundance of beautiful fish. We were in The Rift Valley, 1500 feet above sea level, but we were low compared with the surrounding Central African region, and it was hot throughout most of the year. In the

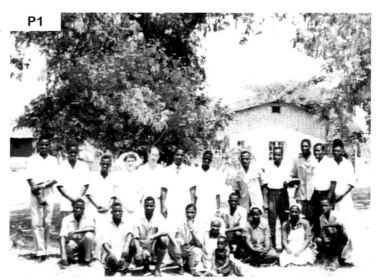

Fort there were government offices, called the Boma, with a district commissioner in the Colonial Service, and three assistant district commissioners, all of whom were university graduates. The small hospital had male and female wards and a maternity wing, and there was an operating theatre which had electricity from the town's generator. The staff consisted of a British sister, an African medical assistant, several African medical aides, and an African midwife, plus the doctor, all seen in picture P1. There was a small club, with a concrete tennis court, a snooker table

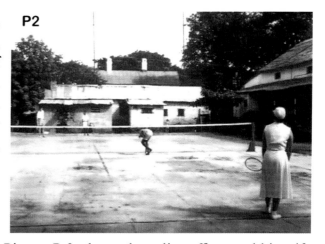

with a rather worn cloth, and a different sort of bar. Picture P 2. shows the police officer and his wife playing tennis in the cool of an early Sunday morning. 100 yards from the hospital compound was my house, seen in picture P 3 with me and my car, a big double storey affair, gauzed in against mosquitoes. Fort Johnston had been the headquarters of the Royal Navy on the lake before the Great War, and the club, the oldest in the country, had been their club. My house had probably housed the officers. The first naval engagement in the war was successfully made by the Royal Navy in 1914, when their gunboat put out of action the German one on the other side of the lake. The news of the outbreak of war had not reached Tanganyika until after the engagement.

The 'garden' at the back of my house ran down to the Shire where crocs and hippos abounded. I never saw them but heard the hippos each night when they foraged and splashed around making their terrible grunts and bellows at the bottom of the garden. I gave hospitality one night to a small family passing through the Fort and told them not to be worried about the hippo noises. I could imitate the double noise quite well and gave them an example. The parents slept in the room next to mine, and in between was a small connecting room where their little girl slept. In the night the hippos obliged beautifully, and I heard the little girl say 'Mummy, was that Dr Gilchrist?'

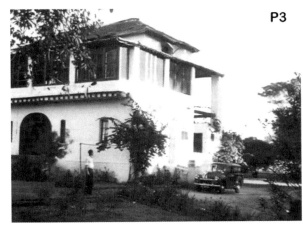

P3

P4

Picture P 4 shows the river Shire at the bottom of my 'garden', while P 5 shows the upstairs verandah which was my living room. Note the shorts and the naughty pipe and tobacco tin.

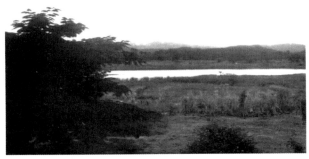

We did not eat well at the Fort, at least I as a bachelor did not. My servant made the bread, and the paraffin fridges struggled to keep cool the milk made from powder. I lost weight and on two occasions was admitted to Zomba hospital eighty miles away, first in 1957 with hepatitis and later with severe diarrhoea and vomiting.

P5

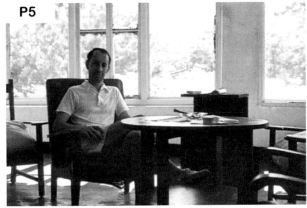

The Fort Johnston District was large, probably the largest in the country with an area of about 3000 square miles, a little larger than Hampshire and Wiltshire combined, and I was the only doctor. There were seven dispensaries scattered in all directions, each with a medical aide in charge and stocked up with medicines, three of them being 60 miles away from the Fort. See diagram D 3 taken from my earlier book which shows the positions of the dispensaries. Eventually, I visited them all in turn each Friday by Land Rover. The medical aides knew when it was their turn and kept aside the patients they wanted me to see. Those needing hospital treatment came back with me, and sometimes we returned with the Land Rover packed full, in the dark.

D3

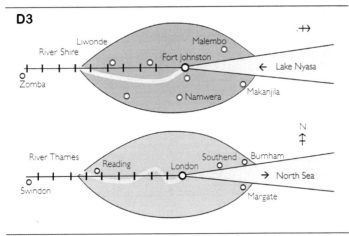

Picture 12: The Fort Johnston district showing my seven dispensaries, and a region in Southern England of the same area.

Originally, I suppose, the doctors in the Colonial Service would have been the first teachers of those men who wished to join the medical service. Then some of those who had been taught and learned by experience, may have passed on their knowledge to some of the next generation of doctors, and doctors and medical assistants would teach one another. For example, all my major operations were conducted under open ether, dropped on a Schimmelbusch mask, after induction with ethyl chloride spray. I learned how to do this from the medical assistants.

Towards the end of 1956, I began to prepare for Christmas. I bought sweets and cigarettes for the patients and decided to have a party for the staff. I drove a long way over to P.E.A., (Portuguese East Africa, now Mozambique), and bought a large turkey. We fattened it up and it was ready on the table on Christmas Day. All the staff were present in my house, and I had a nice bottle of sherry to serve, when I was called away to the hospital. When I returned, the Land Rover driver and the Lab assistant were nodding off to sleep with pleasant looks on their faces, and the sherry bottle was empty.

Those in the Colonial Service had to pass the appropriate level of the indigenous language examination before being promoted. For example, an assistant district commissioner had to pass the advanced written and spoken parts of the Cinyanja exam before being promoted to District Commissioner, while a road supervisor need only pass the lower grade.

In the Federal Service the language exams were dropped, but I wanted to learn the local language and talk with my patients. I arranged for Mr Kumsinda, our medical assistant, to teach me Cinyanja, the language of the country. He came into my house each week and covered the subject comprehensively. Silas Kumsinda was a very good man. We became friends. I recommended him for promotion, and he became a successful senior medical assistant. In the first picture he is standing on my left.

I must confess that the work that I enjoyed most was the major surgery, especially some of the acute emergency cases if we were able to save them. The medical assistants could cope with the medical cases, but the surgery required a doctor with the necessary anatomical knowledge and interest in the subject. I was well qualified to do the work; anatomy was my favourite subject, and I had been given a certificate of merit after the anatomy course at the Middlesex. Also, the lecture course at the Royal College and my study of the lungs, plus my pathology year at Nottingham, the six months' accidents at Birmingham, and the year's light work in the lab in Bulawayo where I had already begun again to prepare for the exams of the Royal College, made me a suitable candidate. I did so much surgery, it is difficult to choose what to relate. There were Caesarean sections, ruptured uteruses, inguinal hernias, intestinal obstructions, chronic osteomyelitis, crocodile and hippo bites, puff adder bites and fractures. We had no blood, no x-rays, no mobile phones, and no HIV. Sewing up after an intestinal obstruction without muscle relaxants, (I learned to use them later), could be the longest part of the operation. Some of the cases were overwhelmingly challenging, but something had to be done. I had to plunge in, with the reassurance that if they weren't tackled, they might all die.

I experimented with anaesthetics. I wondered why we had to induce with ethyl chloride spray, and I tried once without it. Instead of the patient going under smoothly, she and the medical assistant went up and down and round the operating table in a long, big struggle before she finally succumbed. I did not try it again. I tried chloroform, quite the best anaesthetic I had used. It gave a smooth induction without a struggle, and adequate depth of anaesthesia for major surgery, but I did not persist with it because I knew it could damage the liver. The Schimmelbusch mask was not ideal, especially for those patients who had lost a lot of blood, because it reduced the outflow of carbon-dioxide and the inflow of oxygen. I did several of my inguinal hernias under local anaesthesia.

Mango trees abounded by the lake shore, and when the fruits were in season the children would climb up and pick them. Some children fell down and broke their bones, they were known as mango fractures. The unripe fruits were very fibrous and indigestible. A strong young man from P.E.A., came in with intestinal obstruction. I took him into theatre and removed a large kidney dish full of impacted mango fibre from his small intestine.

Then there was my first hysterectomy, which took me three hours. During a ward round I came across a woman lying quietly in bed, with a large swelling which occupied nearly all of her abdomen. In theatre it was difficult. I did not want to cut the ureters, and I couldn't see anything behind or below because of the lump. I went slowly and eventually it came out. It was a large fibroid uterus. Then my theatre assistant told me she was his mother! Now her son was twenty-one, and he was her only child, and she had not lactated for twenty-one years. But after the operation she made up for that and began to produce milk. Not watery milk, but rich full cream milk. It went on for many weeks, even though she had no baby to suckle. I could not understand it, I knew nothing of the physiology of lactation. But later, having delved into the subject, it was as if she had been pregnant for many years, and her uterus may have secreted oestrogen and progesterone which are secreted by the placenta in pregnancy, and which inhibit the secretion of prolactin by the anterior pituitary. In which case, the hysterectomy would have been the equivalent of the separation of the placenta in a normal delivery, with the cancellation of the inhibition and subsequent onset of lactation. But why did the milk continue to flow? Had the prolactin system been suppressed for so long, that there had been a compensatory increase in the development of that part of the anterior pituitary? I will leave it to the experts to decide, those in endocrinology and others who specialise in the cause of tumours.

We rescued every ruptured uterus which reached us, but there was one I was unable to save. On a morning ward round a most terrible shriek came from the labour ward. I hastened over and saw a fine-looking pregnant woman dead on the delivery couch. She must have ruptured. We put her body in the boot of my car, and I took her home to her village which lay off the beaten track some twenty miles away and handed her over to her sad husband.

Two of the Caesars died after I had successfully delivered the babies. The uteruses may have been in a pre-ruptured condition because they tore badly and bled heavily as I was repairing them. They were put on intravenous fluids and sent to the ward, where the night medical aide was instructed to tell me if they were not well. He did not do this, only saying in the morning that they had died in the night. When we had a third case like this, I seated the medical aide at the foot of her bed, and I lay down on the bed next to hers. I gave him strict instructions to take her pulse every fifteen minutes and wake me every thirty minutes so that I could check the blood pressure. But he went to sleep, and I was waking him up! She survived and I never lost another Caesar. The first time I had slept with a woman.

In hindsight, I may have been wrong to give intravenous fluids when there was no blood available. It may have kept the blood pressure up and increased the blood loss. Now I see the value of giving morphia, which may settle the patient, lower the blood pressure, and reduce bleeding. Again, in hindsight, I was negligent in not sterilising every Caesarean section and every ruptured uterus. The next pregnancy may end in rupture.

I came across a few cases of chronic osteomyelitis, with holes or sinuses in the shaft of the infected bone discharging pus. Covering the shaft of the bone was new bone known as involucrum, with gaps in it which allowed the pus to escape from the sinuses. I had seen several examples preserved in jars in the John Hunter Museum in 1953. I treated them by first removing the involucrum, then chiselling off the shaft in layers until I came down to heathy bleeding bone, and packed the exposed raw bone with flavine gauze and left the wound open. They all healed well.

Some of our babies were born with congenital malformations, three of them seen here, in P 6 with a cleft lip, P 7 with ectopia vesicae, the bladder opening onto the front of the abdomen, and P 8 with amelia, having no arms. I repaired the cleft lips as best I could. Nothing could be done for the others.

At the end of 1957. I took home leave and lived with my parents, staying for three weeks in the guest wing of East Grinstead hospital and watched the surgeons performing their plastic surgery. I did not see a cleft lip repaired but attended a lecture on the subject and made careful notes. The theatre sister gave me a list of the instruments I would need, and I was able to buy them and take them back to the Fort.

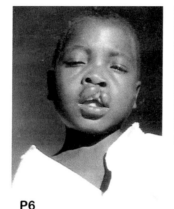

P6

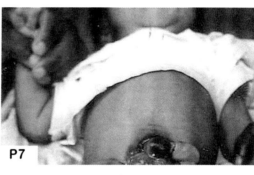

P7

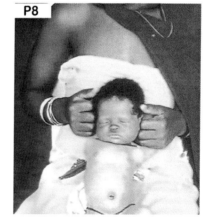

P8

The officer in charge of medical stores in Zomba, was able to get me an M.R.C. Grey wedge haemoglobinometer, and we checked the haemoglobin levels on our hospital patients weekly. All our patients were anaemic. Again, I asked Zomba for Imferon, and it was imported for me. I put the adults on iron pills daily and children on syrup. Those adults with less than 50% haemoglobin were given one injection each week, and those with less than 20% were given an injection twice a week. The results were interesting, whichever route used, injection pills or syrup, all the patients improved by 10% each week. Imferon became popular, but iron injections were unnecessary, except for those patients we lost track of who would have had a depot of iron to continue the treatment.

The U.M.C.A. (Universities Mission to Central Africa) Bishop at Mponda, three miles from the Fort, asked me to circumcise forty of his proselytes, who were secluded in a palisaded compound in the bush somewhere. I took three of my senior medical aides to the place with all the necessary equipment, divided us into two teams and showed them how it was done under local anaesthesia. One of us gave the local and the other operated. I operated on ten, then handed over to my partner to do the next ten, with me giving the anaesthetic. I kept an eye on the other team, one doing the surgery on ten boys, then the other taking over to do the rest. We finished the forty that morning and were invited to lunch with the Bishop at his Mponda headquarters.

I was on my way to one of our dispensaries, and I was waved down by its medical aide. A young woman was having difficulties in labour. He led me to her hut, and when I had adapted to the gloom in the hut I could see the woman on the ground with her mother kneeling beside her. With some reassurance from me and cooperation from her, the baby was slowly delivered, with relief for all of us in the hut. The mother then produced a large square of bark cloth, cut off a small piece and placed it over the baby's cut umbilical cord. The medical aide described the local custom for a firstborn child. The bark is cut from a baobab tree. A piece is used to cover the navel, and another piece cleans the baby's bottom. The rest swaddles the baby, and when it has been used up the baby is weaned. I had often seen the depressed scars on the trees from where the bark had been cut.

That medical aide was one of my best. He died from oesophageal cancer. He was relatively young and a cigarette smoker. It was the second time I had met that condition. The first one had been my own grandfather, whom I had seen dying in Tunbridge Wells Hospital in 1936, with a feeding tube in his stomach. He was about seventy years old, and a pipe smoker, and the little Sussex village of Etchingham lost the skills of its carpenter. I remember saying to him 'Good luck Grandad,' as I shook his hand.

I witnessed other customs in the Fort; I remember one because of my love of music. From my upstairs verandah I could see what went on in the hospital compound. I often saw the wives pounding their maize in the hollowed-out tree trunks with a heavy pole. 'Ku sinja ndi munsi', to pound with a pole. Sometimes there would be two women pounding in the same trunk, and on one occasion there were three, all taking it in turns and singing to the rhythm. Sometimes one of the women with a large tummy would be absent for a day, re-appearing the next day with a slimmer figure and a little bundle on her back to rejoin the others. 'Music while you work.'

I saw several cases of tetanus, none of them serious, without convulsions or trismus. I thought it was a mild disease.

A missionary couple arrived from their station 60 miles away on the lake shore, with their large dog carrying a partly delivered dead puppy. It had been a breech delivery with extended neck and face anterior, and the head arrested at the pelvis. It was a simple thing to do, I twisted the head round with the face posterior, hooked a finger in its mouth, flexing the head, and extracted it easily.

There was plenty of wildlife in the district, though I was more interested in the people. I have already mentioned the unseen crocs and hippos. Occasionally there were leopard footprints near my house, and once a lion came through the ground at night. The lion's growl started on a high note and came down low, while the hyena's cry began low and ended in a shrill high crescendo. Baboons were fairly common, and roamed around in families, parents, and children. The senior ones were big heavy animals.

There was a lot of bird life on the lake. I saw Nkwazi the fish eagle, with its black and white plumage and characteristic cry, catch its prey. There were many cormorants. After diving for fish, they would sit drying themselves with their wings held out sideways like scarecrows. I came across a flock of guinea fowl feeding on the ground. I got out of my car to have a closer look, but they took to the air and came for me at eye level like a squadron of spitfires, and I jumped back into my car-quickly. They may taste nice on the table but are not very friendly before they are cooked.

I saw a variety of snakes. Returning to the Fort at dusk in the Land Rover with Mr. Kumsinda, he said 'oh a big snake.' I drove on. Then this quietly spoken gentleman said, 'In all my life I have never seen such a big snake.' I slammed on the brakes and reversed. Our back wheels were lifted off the road with a b-bump as the back wheels first struck the snake then the road behind it, then the front wheels with another b-bump. We had run over this creature as it was crossing the dirt road, and now we could see it, a huge, long thick serpent in coils, stretched across the road. It gave me such a nasty look as it slithered off into the bush at the side of the road. The villagers on either side of the road leading from the Fort kept a lot of sheep and goats. I assumed they were the serpent's staple diet. They were our diet too. When our health assistant was away inspecting the villages, I had to inspect the meat before it could be sold. The goat and sheep meat was very lean and tasted about the same to me. Sometimes I would drive off to the Palm Beach Inn, nine miles away on the lake shore, and have a good meal of fried lake fish, especially on a Sunday for lunch. The alternative was to eat in my lonely dining room, as quickly as possible.

Early in 1959 there was political unrest in the country. On a few occasions I had met Henry Chipembere (Rhinocerus), who was one of the three lieutenants who had brought Dr Banda back to Nyasaland. He invited me to a gathering to hear what Dr Banda had to say. It was on a Sunday morning in the open air, though some of us were provided with chairs. Banda was most derogatory and rude about the Federation and his white guests, and his views were quite the opposite of my own, and after half an hour of insults I got up and left. Henry Chipembere protested strongly as I passed him at the end of the row, but I made my excuses and went to Palm Beach, where the atmosphere was more cordial, and the lunch delicious.

There was tension in the air, you could feel it. On 3rd March 1959 a state of emergency was declared. One morning to our relief, 120 young Rhodesian soldiers were walking round the Fort in pairs with fixed bayonets. We relaxed. The troops were billeted in the sisters' vacant house. The district sisters had been posted to Blantyre to staff the new Queen Elizabeth Hospital. The troops left us and moved up country.

With my gardener and another man I employed, they began to landscape the surrounds of my house, first to terrace the garden, then to build a path at the side leading down to the river, where in future I might keep a boat. I stood at the end of the path and looked up stream and down, and contemplated things. Perhaps it had been like this for five hundred years and could be the same for the next five hundred. I continued in thought. 'This is my home, where I want to spend the rest of my life.' But it was not to be.

Sometimes we saw cases of acute mania when the patient would scream and act violently. We sedated them with injections of paraldehyde and sent them to the Zomba mental hospital under police escort. The doctor in charge of the hospital had recently been replaced by a psychiatrist, who had other ideas and stopped us from sending such patients to him. He sent us a circular describing how to treat them with largactil. When the next such patient arrived, he was treated in this way and was shut up in a side room. I told the medical aide to call me if the treatment did not work. In the early hours of the next morning the patient was screaming, and I waited to be called, but the medical aide did not come. At last, I got of bed and went to the ward. The medical aide was sitting calmly on the steps outside the ward and chatting to a friend. I told him he was useless and incompetent. Later that morning there was a knock on my door. When I said, 'Come in', about ten of my staff came in and surrounded me. The ringleader said, 'Did you say he was useless and incompetent.' I was visibly shaken and did not reply. They would not leave my office. I managed to get to the phone and told the A.D.C. what was happening, and he contacted the P.M.O. (provincial medical officer) in Blantyre. I went to my house and had a cup of tea. I was very upset and worried. The PMO arrived after some hours and listened to them as they harangued about me quite inaccurately, (i.e. Lies). I left them to it. When the PMO came out, he did not come over to me to ask my side of the story, but with the staff looking on he gave me a nod, climbed into his car, and drove off. I had to see the DMS, (Director of Medical Services), who also did not ask my side of the story, but said I been in the Fort too long and posted me to Blantyre. It was some time before I was able to leave, and those last few weeks were very difficult for me. On the morning of my departure, I scratched my initials on a baobab tree in the garden, and a visiting priest took this picture, P 9, as I stood in front of the tree.

P 10 shows the Canadian de Havilland, which gave the Fort a weekly service from Blantyre. Note the fire-fighting equipment.

That unpleasant incident at Fort Johnston taught me a great deal. I learned a lot about some of my staff, more about the PMO, something of the DMS, and even the psychiatrist, it gave me a glimpse of him too. But most of all it taught me about myself, how I had reacted badly in a potentially dangerous situation. It caught me unawares, I was scared and showed it. Next time, if there is a next time, I will act with calmness (I hope), like the cats who carry on scratching or licking themselves as if there is nothing to worry about.

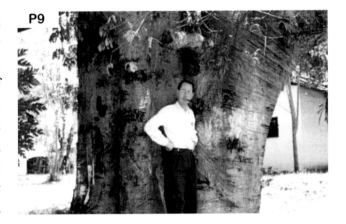

P9

P10

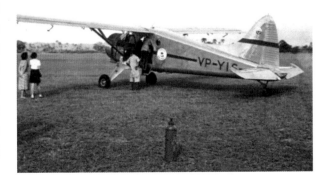

I was very sorry to leave Fort Johnston, it had been my first venture into African Africa, and I had chosen it myself. I had often thought it takes three months to learn a job, but this one took three years. And just when I thought everything was going well, and that I would settle down there, I was suddenly plucked out of it unceremoniously. Those three years were very special for me, that sort of job is not so easily obtained now, with improved communications and the shrinking world. I will always be grateful that I was able to be part of a special experience. I could never forget the Fort.

There were several districts in Nyasaland, each with its own doctor meeting the challenging work in a part of Africa far from his own country. The first Secretary for Health was Richard Morris. When he died Professor Michael Gelfand, an expert on African diseases and customs, wrote an obituary in the Central Africa Medical Journal. He said, 'Richard Morris created the finest medical service in Africa.'

Blantyre.

I worked in the newly built Queen Elizabeth Hospital, a large sprawling affair, where the Canadian matron did her rounds on a bicycle. I was put in charge of an adult male ward. One of the patients had been savaged by a leopard. He had killed the animal with his bare hands, but the front of his body had been gouged terribly. He lay in his bed for many weeks and was eventually allowed to go home with his scars. I thought he deserved a medal. The Medical Superintendent was a large friendly Scot who had a surgical degree. He taught me endotracheal intubation and the use of muscle relaxants. I also learned how to do the lower segment Caesarean section, which was an improvement on the classical method I had used at the Fort, and which would prove to be of benefit for my future Caesareans sections. We had x-rays, and a laboratory, with a pathologist in charge who was a cheerful contemporary of mine from the same medical school. When he and the superintendent bumped into each other, you could hear their laughter two corridors away.

For three weeks, I was posted from Blantyre to Mlanje, a small station where the doctor was leaving for South Africa. He had arranged for all the emergency obstetric work to be taken over by the dedicated doctor at a nearby mission, and my stay there was a holiday. The senior medical assistant was my friend Silas Kumsinda who had taught me Cinyanja at the Fort. He trebled the attendances at Mlanje hospital. I palled up with the young police officer and his wife. We played snooker at the club, and on one Saturday afternoon we walked up to the first level of magnificent Mount Mlanji. Shortly after my return to Blantyre I was Posted to Dedza in the Central Province. I had spent six easy months away from district work and I had picked up some useful medical knowledge too. The Fort Johnston wounds were already healing, and I was beginning to see the benefit of a change I had not asked for. Without doubt the DMS had been correct in moving me from the Fort. I remember him with gratitude.

Dedza.

Dedza was the antithesis of Fort Johnston. It was a small station high up in the cool Angoni Highlands of the Central Province on the western side of the lake. In the short winter months, we had fires in our homes. The houses were not supplied with electricity, and we used paraffin pressure lamps for illumination. The postmaster had secretly connected the post-office generator to our hospital theatre, and we always had lights there. The Angoni and Achewa staff were friendly and respectful, and we got on well. They spoke Cinyanja nicely, and I was able to resume my study of the language. On 24th March 1960 I passed the oral and written parts of the advanced examination. I introduced my method of visiting the clinics monthly. There were fewer than at the Fort and they were nearer the hospital.

This picture, P 11, of the Dedza staff, brings back the fondest memories of my work in Africa. I remember them all, but only the names of those who worked closest to me. The medical assistant on my right is Mr. Mpekansambo. His wife is in the pink uniform next to him. On her right is a man of mixed race, an enthusiastic young gentleman, and on his right, the man wearing the fez, is the hospital messenger. Chilabade, my able theatre assistant in his gown is on my left, and further back between us is Mr, Sikoya, my loyal efficient hospital secretary. A happy family.

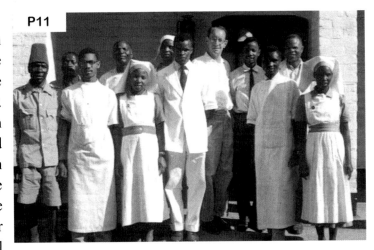

P11

We began to see ruptured ectopic pregnancies in Dedza, about one a month. I had seen none in the Fort, and for the first time I had to deal with this important obstetric emergency. The patient had missed a period, then had sudden abdominal pain and a discharge of blood. Without delay we took her to theatre, anaesthetised her and opened her abdomen. It was full of blood, nothing else could be seen. I plunged in, drew up the uterus and clamped the ruptured tube and removed it. One of our early cases with a rupture in the left tube, returned later with another. Again, I plunged in and removed the right tube. But the ectopic had implanted itself on the stump of the left tube, and I had sterilised her. With so many cases I soon got the hang of it, and we saved them all except one. During the emergency, the doctor at Ncheu, some 40 miles to the south of us had been posted to Nkata Bay and I covered his station. One evening the medical assistant at Ncheu phoned us and said he had an ectopic pregnancy. We asked him to send her over quickly, and we prepared the theatre. But they came very late, she had bled white, and died on the table as I opened her abdomen, full of her lost blood.

Months later, when I had left Dedza, the Ncheu doctor had returned to his station, and he was covering Dedza. I had left him an undiagnosed ectopic pregnancy which turned out to be an abdominal pregnancy. He delivered the baby successfully by Caesarean section. It must have been a rare experience when the amniotic fluid gushed out as he opened the abdomen to reveal a live baby outside the uterus. He left the placenta on the posterior abdominal wall where it had attached itself. He wrote up this case in our monthly newsletter. The doctor was of mixed African and Indian race, highly respected by all in Ncheu. I believe he became the first professor of obstetrics in the new Malawi.

I had not been long in Dedza when the health assistant reported smallpox in one of the villages. The doctor had to report each case to Medical H.Q. by telegram, after having seen the case personally. We did not move the patients, and the doctor had to go to the village, which in this case was a large one which straddled the border with P.E.A., and on my first visit I saw fifty-six cases. We treated them with antibiotics. On my next visit I had my camera and took photos of some of the patients. Two of them P 12, and P 13, show the girls with the rash, while the third P 14, shows a later healed stage known locally as Ntomba.

(I would have been working in Dedza in 1960. On the 26th of October 1979, the World Health Organisation eradicated smallpox from the world.)

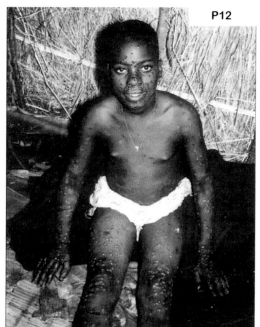

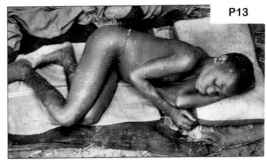

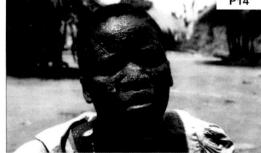

The hospital cook brought his son to me with a large hare lip on the right side. I revised the East Grinstead lecture, took him to theatre and intubated him through the nose, while the anaesthetic was intravenous pentothal. I took several pictures afterwards, but had taken none before, so I reversed the earlier left sided in P15 one, to show you what the pre-op condition would have looked like.

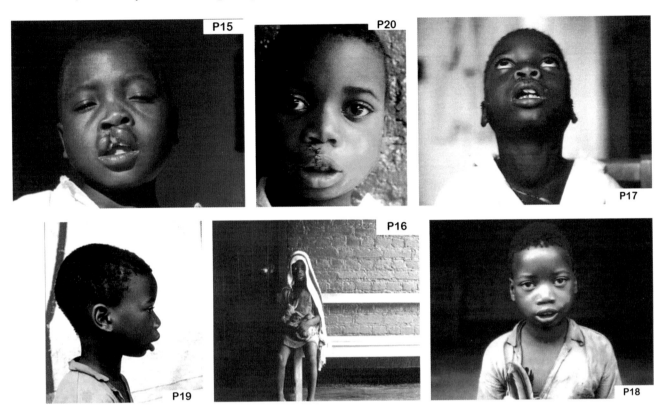

I have changed the order of the pictures to show the correct time sequence when they were taken. P 20 was the first picture taken shortly after the operation. The sutures were removed shortly afterwards, probably no later than five days after the operation, and I would have supported the wound with a strip of plaster for a day or two later, to reduce scarring from the sutures. P17. Pictures 20, 17, and 19, show the importance of removing the correct amount of lip, and ensuring that the new lip is not stretched across the face, otherwise it will look ugly and show that an attempt has been made to repair a hare lip. Note the wider right nostril in P 17, and the right eye in P 16 and P 20, displaced to the side, which show that the fault in facial development had spread upwards beyond the lip and teeth. P 16 shows him waiting outside my office with a chicken he brought me, and P 18 gives a closer view of him with the chicken. A happy grateful boy.

Shortly afterwards a young man appeared with an ugly double cleft lip. I took pictures and took him to theatre, broke the upper gums, the maxillae, with a blunt instrument, pushed them back into place and repaired the lip as best I could. The result was not perfect but an improvement. P's 21-24. When he came back later, he told me he had got married.

The Federal government had given each of the three territories an A level boarding school for African students. In

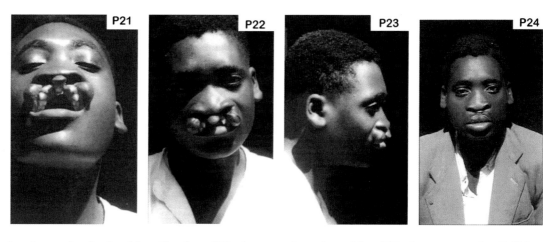

Nyasaland the school was in the healthy district of Dedza, on the other side of Dedza mountain. I did not visit the school but treated some of the students. We admitted one of them who was very ill. The laboratory assistant showed me a tube of his blood which was almost completely haemolysed, leaving the red cells at the bottom of the tube below the clear serum. I was powerless to help him, and he died of blackwater fever, the only case I had seen, in an African student in high up healthy Dedza.

One night the medical assistant sent the messenger to me with a note telling me there was a ruptured uterus in the hospital and he could hear the foetal heart. I dashed to the hospital and delivered a live baby. Part of the placenta was still attached to the torn uterus. Such a rare case. Top marks for the medical assistant, Green Nyrenda, a Tumbuka from the Northern Province.

We had a small club in Dedza, and the club house and two tennis courts were not far from my house. I won the annual men's singles competition and was elected captain. We had an annual competition against Lilongwe, whose members included some strong tobacco farmers with a reputation for tennis we had heard of. I arranged trials to choose our best players. After choosing the team, the D.C.'s wife phoned me. Two of the ladies not chosen were in tears. 'They always played against Lilongwe.' One of them had a flashy serve which never went in. Then she did the same for the second serve with the same result. Nevertheless, I relented and brought them in. We were walloped, especially by their captain who overwhelmed me. Those Lilongwe tobacco farmers were invincible. Perhaps that is what they mostly did-tennis.

The middle-aged pair of the D.C. and his friend challenged me and my partner to a game. We were soon outplaying them. My partner was delivering incredible booming shots across the net, and I was contributing too. We were getting more and more confident as we dominated the game, while Gabe and Ted were throwing themselves all over the place in desperation as the balls whistled past. 'Yours Gabe, no yours Ted,' they were shouting to each other, encouragingly, pleadingly, hopefully, as they ballerina-ed towards and away from each other, with their rackets just swishing the air. A better imitation of the dancing animals in Fantasia's 'Dance of the hours' I had not seen, and I was soon contorted with laughter. I collapsed on the ground completely useless with tears running down my face, and the game came to an end.

We had a small golf course in Dedza with sand greens. (You used a wooden scraper before putting). There were two tees for each hole, which made it into an 18- hole course. It intrigued me, and after the tennis tears, I decided to try my hand at golf. I bought four clubs from someone, a 2, a 5, an 8 iron and a putter, borrowed Ben Hogan's wonderful little book 'Power Golf' and devoured it. I practised my swing daily. A year later, after buying a driver, my handicap was 12 and I began to love the game more than tennis.

Towards the end of 1960, I was asked if I would like to relieve the Northern Province PMO for three months. He was taking his daughter to America for an open-heart operation. I accepted readily. Before I left, during an operation, Chilabade said 'So you are on the ladder.' I had had no ambitions to climb it, but the offer sounded attractive, and I was soon on my way further up north to Mzuzu, the Provincial Capital.

Eventually, my move from Fort Johnston had been beneficial, but the way it happened left me shocked and disappointed. My move from Dedza was quite the opposite, and I left cheerfully. Dedza had been a reward for me, a compensation for the humiliation I had suffered at the Fort. The District, The Climate, The Work and The Staff, where I passed the language exam and learned to play golf. In no other job, before or since, was I as happy as I had been in Dedza.

Mzuzu.

I drove to Mzuzu, the provincial capital, and threw myself into the job. The journey up was interesting. After passing Kasungu, eighty miles north of Lilongwe, the climate changed. The air was moister, and the scrub land gave way to wooded country. We were equatorial, the 10- degree south latitude cut across the northern tip of Nyasaland, which included the little township of Karonga near the lake shore.

Shortly after arriving in Mzuzu, I had a call from the doctor in Karonga. One of his staff was being intimidated by the local people. I drove up straight away and spent Christmas with the doctor and his wife. It was a difficult time for some of our federal employees during the emergency, and some of the people up north were very belligerent. I think my meeting with the intimidated man helped to reassure him. I visited Karonga twice more, on each occasion flying up in the Canadian Beaver, and less than two years after my undignified exit from the Fort, I was flying round the Northern Province as the PMO.

There was development in Mzuzu, I had a new house. There were even some shops, and I fed well, especially on Australian lamb which arrived deep frozen. I ran a small clinic from my house. On two occasions I visited the doctor at Mzimba on the other side of the forested high Vipya plateau. I visited Nkata Bay each week, and sometimes went further on down to Chinteche, driving through the government experimental rubber plantation on the way. Chinteche was an interesting place. In the rainy season it would be cut off by a swollen river and the medical assistant had to do the Caesars. The staple diet was not maize (chimanga), but cassava (chinangwa). While I was in Mzuzu, elections were held to vote in the new government, which was won by the Malawi Congress Party, and the Federation was to be dissolved on the last day of 1963. Before I had left Dedza, I had been asked by medical H.Q. what my plans were. I had replied 'This is a Nicer Land, but there is the Road Easier,' and towards the end of the Federation I was offered the post of medical superintendent of Fort Victoria hospital in Southern Rhodesia.

At the end of my three months in the north, I did not return to Dedza, I was asked to take over Lilongwe Hospitals as Medical Officer in charge. My work in the rural areas seemed to have come to an end, after having spent almost five years there. It had been a privilege for me to practise the widest spectrum of medical and surgical conditions during that time, which had taught me more than I could have imagined.

Caesars, ruptured uteruses, ectopic pregnancies. *Blood loss, that is what I had to deal with, acute, from the genital tract of the African ladies, and chronic, from malnutrition and tropical diseases, especially in those who lived near the lake shore.*

Lilongwe.

The European and African hospitals in Lilongwe were the third busiest in the Federation after Salisbury and Bulawayo, and we had only three doctors, who were contemporaries of mine. I took over the surgery and the admin, another doctor with the higher qualification of MRCP looked after the medical cases, and the third young doctor, who had had a vast experience in Port Herald on the lower Shire, similar to mine, worked in the maternity unit. We had an x-ray machine and a lady to work it. We were now working in a town, and in the middle of it was an eighteen-hole golf course. Things were always happening in Lilongwe, the first occurred to me soon after I arrived there. Returning late from a court case in Blantyre, I was assaulted by a thug who knocked me out unconscious. When I woke up, I drove to Lilongwe police station. The O.C. sent out a message across the country, and my assailant was picked up the next morning at 5 am, after having assaulted two other men in Dedza. My face was stitched up by the PMO, and he advised me to rest for a week. But in the next night a Portuguese lady from Dedza whom I knew, came in with a ruptured ectopic, and I got up and operated on her. Another Dedza ectopic.

I had already arranged a family reunion with my sister and her husband from New Zealand, and on arriving at Heathrow I told them about the assault because I had to have an operation on my nose. Janet said, 'Don't tell Mum and Dad,' and I didn't. But later, sitting in the garden at home, my mother, looking very concerned, drew up a chair and sat close to me, and told me how, a few weeks ago, she had sat up in the middle of the night and woken my father and said, 'Something has happened to Alan.' I then told her about the assault. I had the operation on my nose. The septum was removed, and I looked like a boxer or rugby player who had had the same sort of operation.

A fine young African doctor joined us, accompanied by his wife and two children. He had qualified from Fort Hare University in South Africa. He entertained me in his house with singing and guitar playing. He joined me in theatre and showed me how to treat a fractured shaft of femur with an intra-medullary nail. He had seen it done in Salisbury. I gave him half my outpatient clinics. Ther was no problem with the African or Asian, but the local white farmers objected when it came to the European. I was confronted in my office by two of the farmers who had beaten us at tennis, and a group of officials from medical headquarters in Salisbury. I had to rescind my arrangement, and our fourth doctor was posted to Port Herald on the lower Shire. He later became a successful pathologist with his own laboratory in Harare.

I did my only white Caesar in Lilongwe, noted not for the colour of her skin, but because it was the first and only time that I had opened the bladder. I stitched it up and we put in a catheter, and the patient was charming about it. But one of the sisters objected strongly when I described my mistake in the notes which were clearly visible in the duty room frequented by staff and patients alike. (The sisters had been responsible for emptying the bladder before the operation). I relented, turned the notes round so that my error was not seen and kept everyone happy.

We were paid a visit by a team of three from Makerere in Uganda led by an English surgeon Denis Burkitt, who were investigating the distribution of a strange tumour which affected the facial skeleton of

African children. I had seen such cases on a ferry crossing the Shire at Liwonde 47 miles down from the Fort. Denis Burkitt's work in Africa, which showed the tumours to result from the double infection of malaria and the Epstein-Barr virus, contributed, I believe, to our understanding of the cause of cancer. The tumour became known as Burkitt's Lymphoma.

There was a training school in Lilongwe for female medical aides, and the doctors helped with the lectures. In my first lecture, the sister in charge, who was the wife of the doctor with the Membership, came in with the trainees and sat behind them. I began by telling them about my treatment of anaemia in Fort Johnston. When I said the injections were unnecessary the sister blurted out 'Blathers.' I explained that they had been my own observations. 'Blathers.' She said again rudely. The lecture broke up in disarray. Later, she and her husband were posted to Northern Rhodesia where he probably became the medical specialist.

When I was trying to repair a fractured skull, the theatre sister showed me some Horsley's wax she had on her tray. She had seen other doctors use it to stop the bleeding from the skull diploe. At that time, I knew nothing of Victor Horsley who had introduced the wax. But I have since read about this remarkable doctor, who was a British surgeon who had been knighted, and who had gained many honours for his pioneer work. He volunteered for service in Mesopotamia during the first world war, and died from the heat in Amarah, Iraq, where he lies buried.

On one of my ward rounds, I met the Karonga ambulance driver, lying in wait for me. He had a large swelling in his upper abdomen. In theatre it proved to be a huge swelling of the right adrenal. The theatre sister worked with me for five and a quarter hours before we removed it successfully. On my ward round the next morning the ward sister said he had died in the night. I thought of two possible reasons, abrupt withdrawal of adrenal secretions, and, more likely, bleeding from arteries poorly ligated when I was tired at the end the operation. The last part of the operation had involved removing the tumour from the descending aorta, with the connecting arteries being very short. I had used catgut, I should have used silk and made certain the vessels were securely ligated. I often think of Hippocrates, he is always reminding me, 'Life is short, Art is long, Judgement difficult,' But judgement depends on experience, and I had had none of adrenal tumours attached to the aorta. Meanwhile, I had left a sad widow and children mourning for the man I had killed. Should I have operated? Sending him to Blantyre or Salisbury was not an option, and Cape Town, where they might have investigated first, was out of the question in those days. Just that one important tragic error I had made, or was it the loss of secretions? Either way, it was the operation which had killed him.

My last story from Lilongwe concerns David Gomile, the young son of an African police officer who had jumped into a rubbish pit, not knowing that the ashes underneath were glowing hot. Both legs were badly burned, and despite all our efforts to save him he continued to lose condition and go downhill. He was not fit enough to have grafts taken from himself, which would have increased the fluid loss. During my stay in East Grinstead, I learned that grafts taken from a close relative could survive for up to six or eight weeks. So, we took him and his mother to theatre, anaesthetised both on either side of me and I took large grafts from her legs. I cut them up into several pieces postage stamp size and applied them to his raw areas. The grafts survived until his own regenerated skin took over and he turned the corner and made a good recovery. Years later, when I was in general practice in Harare, a strong young man walked into my surgery and asked me to repair his contracted tendons on his toes. I had to refuse; I could not do that sort of work. It was David Gomile.

Zomba.

After a year in Lilongwe, I was posted to Zomba, the capital, as Medical Superintendent in charge of the African and European hospitals. At the beginning of the Federation the medical service took over from the Colonial one. At first, I believe, there was some reluctance from the Africans to enter the hospitals, but at the end we couldn't keep them out. The bed occupancy rate in the Zomba African hospital was more than 280%. We had patients on the beds, under the beds and between the beds, and it was all free. There were four of us doctors and sometimes we had a fifth. Although my work was administrative, I did my fair share of the medical work and took it in turns to be on call for emergencies. One evening I had to get up and operate on a ruptured ectopic in the African hospital. At the top hospital I delivered an undiagnosed second twin by pulling down a leg and delivering it feet first. During another evening, the wife of a senior official was in labour, and making no progress in the second stage. I had to find an anaesthetist and do a forceps delivery. The doctor with the best reputation was a captain in the local KAR. (Kings African Rifles), who frequented the local club. I found him at the bar, and he agreed to help. Before she went under, she looked rather horrified at him, but he gave a good anaesthetic, helped by the ethanol fumes during the induction, and the delivery had a successful outcome.

I ran a daily outpatient's clinic in the European hospital. The Federation was coming to an end, and I met some interesting people there. Some were destined to be governors of the remnants of the Empire which still existed in other far-flung places in the world. I also met some of the new African leaders of the country who had been given houses formerly occupied by Europeans. One of them was Henry Chipembere, who was sick, and I had to visit him in his new home. An interesting experience meeting again with the angry man I had last seen in Fort Johnston, and we were having a friendly patient and doctor relationship.

There was an active amateur drama group in Zomba with some talented members. The Minister for Finance put on 'The Yeomen of the Guard.', and I joined in as one of the bearded yeomen. Near me was a lovely young maid in the chorus whose beautiful eyes always seemed to be coming in my direction, and mine in hers I suppose. She shared her sandwiches with me in the interval of the dress rehearsal, and after the public performance I fell madly in love with her. She was Pauline, the daughter of a local farmer and businessman, and had been born in Zomba hospital 21 years previously. We were married the following year on 17th August 1963 in Blantyre. Pauline was 22, and I had just passed my 39th birthday. The priest had forgotten to arrange for an organist, and we walked down the aisle in deathly silence, without Richard Wagner or Felix Mendelssohn. P 25 and P26.

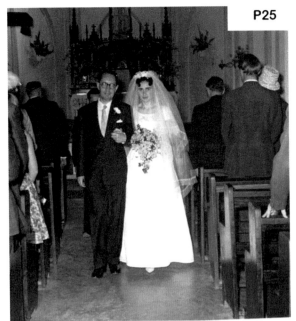

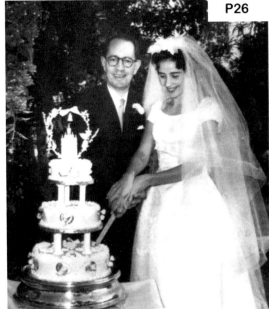

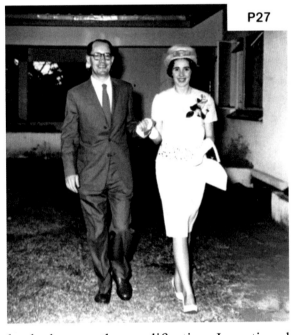

After the reception we left for Fort Victoria in Southern Rhodesia, where I had been offered the post of medical superintendent of the hospital, as I mentioned earlier. We travelled in two cars with my servant and his wife and young son, plus a dog and Pauline's three cats.

Going away to Southern Rhodesia.

My several appointments in Nyasaland deserve a summary. They all took place in a part of Africa I had chosen and loved. Most of my patients had been Africans, who had put their trust in a stranger from England, though often they had had no option. I enjoyed working with them, they were born strong and led lives which developed their strength, but many were afflicted with diseases and malnutrition which took away their strength.

My medical school teaching and post-graduate jobs in England, plus my other qualifications I mentioned earlier, were to prove invaluable in helping me to cope with a wide variety of medical problems in Africa, many of which were life-threatening. It was not too difficult to add the management of tropical diseases to my repertoire, and the district hospital microscopes were often essential for their diagnosis and treatment. I have told you about the blood loss, acute and chronic I had to deal with. I must pay a special tribute to the ladies of Africa who often stoically carry the burden of giving birth under the most difficult conditions. As the multiplicity of conditions continually presented themselves to me, I became more and more competent to deal with them, and the failures, some tragic, grew less and less. I always appreciated the contribution from the medical assistants, they were really the doctors in primary care who sorted out the patients who came to the district hospitals and chose those who needed to see me. But they also kept an eye on the wards and knew what was happening there too. Similarly, the medical aides who manned the dispensaries played a key role in providing a medical service in the most remote parts of the districts. I must stress the benefit of trying to learn the vernacular, how it not only helped me to communicate with my patients, but showed how they appreciated being addressed in their own tongue. Living and working in that part of the world, that part of African Africa, was a special experience for me. The horrors of living in a country wracked by diseases which led many Africans (and Europeans) to a premature grave, were fast disappearing under the efforts of the Federal Ministry of Health, and the whole area, which used to be called British Central Africa, was becoming one of the most healthy and beautiful places on earth.

I always regretted the dissolution of the Federation; did we really have to break it up? When it was dissolved nobody gained, not the white rulers who had designed it, nor the three territories, least of all Malawi. In the seven and a half years I had been in Nyasaland, I had seen around me development everywhere, and I had a vision of the Country on the threshold of a golden era of increasing prosperity. But they rejected it, and it disappeared, possibly for ever. But Zambia and Zimbabwe eventually gained from the damming of the Zambezi at Kariba Gorge, which made Lake Kariba at that time the largest man-made lake in the world, and which would provide unlimited cheap electricity for all time. The lake now appears on all maps of the world, as an epitaph for the Central African Federation of Rhodesia and Nyasaland which had created it, and Africa remains without the finest medical service which had been created by Richard Morris.

Fort Victoria (Now renamed Masvingo)

Fort Victoria was founded in Southern Rhodesia by the Pioneers, who had come up from South Africa in 1890. The altitude was about 3500 feet, and the climate was hot and dry. There was no other town within 200 miles of it. It was at the centre of a cross, Salisbury to the north, Beit Bridge/Messina to the south, Bulawayo to the west and Umtali to the east, and the small white population of about 3000 were a tough, proud, independent resourceful bunch. The hospital was a small affair compared with Zomba. For short periods I had some assistance, but during my four years there I was single-handed for three of them. The TB/Leper hospital at Ngomohuru 35 miles to the south, lost its doctor, and I kept an eye on that as well.

For the major surgery I introduced the techniques I had learned in Blantyre. In the ward the patient would be given injections of pethidine and atropine, and an intravenous drip of saline. In the theatre, the medical assistant injected pentothal into the drip, to be followed by the short-acting muscle relaxant scoline, which paralysed the unconscious patient and stopped him breathing. I then intubated him through the mouth, attached a balloon to the tube and began respirating him with the balloon. I handed over to the medical assistant who continued pumping the balloon and began to give nitrous oxide and oxygen. When I had scrubbed up, I asked the assistant to give the long-acting relaxant flaxedil, which would paralyse the patient throughout the operation to follow. Towards the end of the surgery the assistant reduced the N2O and increased the oxygen, and when I had finished, he gave neostigmine the antidote, which allowed the patient to be sent back to the ward conscious and able to breathe. We used this routine throughout my four years in Fort Victoria without any complications.

I performed a few unusual operations. We admitted a young African boy with congenital hypertrophic pyloric stenosis. He was extremely dehydrated. Large waves of gastric peristalsis could be seen across his abdomen, and the tumour of the pylorus could be felt. Ramstedt's operation was performed, where the hypertrophied pyloric muscle was divided, leaving the mucosa intact, and he rapidly recovered. A woman arrived in obstructed labour with a dead foetus, which I removed by Caesarean section. She had an enormous vesico-vaginal fistula and had lost all the tissues between the bladder and vagina. I transferred the ureters into the colon, and she went home dry. I had attended a lecture on this subject in London, where I heard it would last for ten years. I did no eye surgery, but on two occasions I had to perform a wedge tarsorrhaphy on the inverted lids of entropion, which were scarring the cornea and causing blindness. Very tricky surgery, but the results were worth it. Then one of my favourite operations, remove gangrenous bowel from a strangulated inguinal hernia, perform the anastomosis, replace the bowel in the abdomen and repair the hernia.

From the beginning of my posting to Fort Victoria, I was involved with a huge amount of forensic work for the police, as well as doing all the hospital work, and for four years I became a forensic scientist too. This was new for me; I had done only a couple of post-mortems in Nyasaland. The Victoria Province was large, and all the forensic cases were dealt with by the police in the provincial capital, Fort Victoria, and I was the senior government doctor who had to give the medical evidence. I cast my mind back to Nottingham and remembered how important the forensic cases were and had to be managed by the forensic specialist, and here was I catapulted into that high office without the necessary qualifications or experience. I took the work seriously and even enjoyed it, noting my findings carefully. Each case was referred to the local magistrate, and the more serious cases of murder and rape were later referred to the high 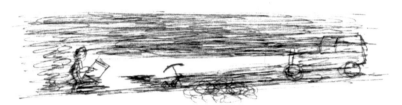 court, which came down to Fort Victoria three times a year. I had a special arrangement with the senior magistrate. I would only be called when it was my turn to enter the witness box, and I need not go home to change into a suit, just attend in my usual working clothes. My work included the collection of human remains from the countryside, night calls for drunken drivers assaults and rape, and post-mortems. The collection of human remains occurred four times, and on each occasion, I was accompanied by the police after work or on the weekends. On two occasions we had to travel a long way to the grave and exhume the body. We started in the daylight but arrived at the grave in the dark. Then the digging began by the police, in the light from the headlights of the police vehicle, reflected down as they went lower, from an aluminium petrol can held by me. See my sketch taken from the first edition of my book. When they arrived at the body, I jumped in and helped to collect the bones. After the court case of the second one, the relatives allowed me to keep the skeleton. It was from the body of a late teenage girl who had died under suspicious circumstances three months earlier. It was a beautiful skeleton with many epiphyses present, which indicated the girl's age. I brought it over when I returned to England and began to write a book about it.

The night calls were frequent and the post-mortems many. I sometimes spent more time in the hospital mortuary than in the wards, and on one day I performed eleven. Four of these were on the Rhodesian table tennis team which had been returning from an international competition in South Africa in a fast car with worn tyres in the rain. On a bend in the road the car rolled, and all were killed. An interesting condition I met there was death from inhaled vomit after drinking too much beer before a fight. My medical assistant, Nicholas told me about the small rapoko seeds which were used in the making of the local beer, and if we cut through the lungs in the post-mortems and saw the terminal bronchi blocked with rapoko and beer, there could be no doubt about the diagnosis of inhaled vomit, and the defendant got off the murder charge.

I often opened the abdomen of a live person in the morning, and a dead one in the afternoon, never the same one, I might add, and if I had forgotten what the internal human viscera looked like, I could refresh my memory in the smelly mortuary. With the success of the new sugar estates in the Low veldt, and the increasing number of workers from the north who flocked down to work there, there were inter-tribal fights which led to injuries and even murder, and the number of high court visits was increased from three to six times a year. So, you see, I was kept busy. The mortuary did not have a cold room, and flies and bluebottles and maggots would emerge from the corpses. I always had Nicholas with me, who sprayed insecticide round me to keep them away. I sometimes came home with the mortuary smells on my clothing, and there were no sweet kisses from Pauline.

Towards the end of my stay in Fort Victoria, I asked H.Q. for a cold room for the mortuary, but they refused. They never came near in those four years, except once when the minister of Health came down to inspect the hospital, and the D.M.S. came down too. They had no idea of the conditions I worked under. So, I sent them a memorandum headed 'Cannibalism in Fort Victoria.' The maggots would crawl down the legs of the post-mortem table, crawl across the floor and under the door to where the staff quarters were.

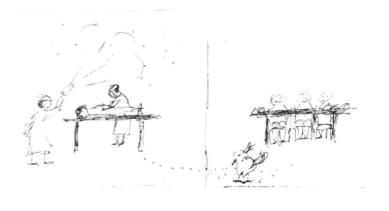

The hens would eat the maggots, and the staff would eat the hens and their eggs. The rotting corpses and the staff were at each end of a food chain. See my other sketch, taken from the first edition of my book. On the day that I left Fort Vic, at the end of May 1967, I saw the foundations of the new cold room being laid. (Later, I understood why we had not had a cold room. Can you guess why? I'll tell you the answer later, when you've had time to think about it).

At the end of April 1965, a baby was delivered in the hospital under my care, and died because we were unable to make her breathe. Her body was taken to the mortuary, where not surprisingly, I was performing a post-mortem for the police. I was engrossed in my work, but my thoughts gradually turned to the body of the little girl. If she had not breathed, would she have been like a foetus which does not breathe in utero, and would her organs still be in the foetal condition? I finished the post-mortem and went over to her and opened the chest. The heart lay horizontally above the raised diaphragm with the unexpanded lungs tucked back on each side. It is a very strange thing, none of the orthodox accounts I have read mentions the raised diaphragm or the horizontal position of the heart. I assume it is the normal arrangement contributing to the economy of space. I removed the heart and lungs together, put them in preserving

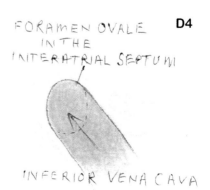

FORAMEN OVALE **D4**
IN THE
INTERATRIAL SEPTUM

INFERIOR VENA CAVA

fluid, took them home and later examined them. Straight away I could see how the streams were separated. It was an emotional moment for me, the first time I had examined a foetal heart which gave me the answer I was seeking. Why had it not been revealed before? I cast my eyes upwards, had I been guided? *The mouth of the inferior vena cava, which was oval, was closely and accurately applied round the foramen ovale in the interatrial wall, and led into the left atrium, not the right, and in life the placental stream would have entered the left atrium directly without having entered the right atrium at all. See D 4.*

This was the first and most precious secret of the foetal circulation. But it had taken a massive political upheaval of part of Africa to move us to Fort Victoria, and to move me into the mortuary where it began to be uncovered. And here was the answer to the riddle I had heard of in the biology class. Each atrium has its own blood supply, arterial for the left and venous for the right, as in the baby. But if the inferior vena cava leads the placental stream into the left atrium, the venous return from the lower body must enter the right atrium by a different route.

Another thing which concerned me was the junction between the aorta and the ductus arteriosus. I had imagined it to be a sort of T junction with the ductus leading into the side of the aorta, because that is how it appeared in all the books I had read. But it is not a T junction, as I found out when examining that little heart. The ductus was a large vessel as large as the aorta and lay side by side with the aorta converging and merging into the descending aorta. See D5. *This is my second secret.* I made accurate drawings of my findings and showed the specimen to Pauline.

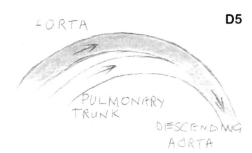

I described these things in the first edition of my book published in Zimbabwe in 2011 and have repeated them in all the next six. I have given copies of some of the later editions to all the British medical schools, so I suppose somebody must have read them. But the old wrong ideas about the two streams of blood entering the foetal right atrium are still being quoted in the latest medical textbooks. However, I am reassured, because they do not seem to have examined foetuses as I have, or taken any pictures or made accurate drawings, just diagrams, or nothing. Why? I have some ideas.

When I was writing the 6th edition of this book, I was able to obtain from the British Institute of Radiology a copy of an article published in the British Journal of Radiology in 1939. It demonstrated with intravascular injections of radio-opaque substances and radiological cinematography the circulation of the blood in live foetal lambs. It revealed the difficult complicated pioneering work performed by A. E. Barclay, Sir Joseph Barcroft, D. H. Barron, and K. J. Franklin, in the Nuffield Institute for Medical Research, Oxford. At that time there was a strict anti-abortion law, with few human foetuses available for research. Only a year earlier, an eminent obstetrician had been arrested by the police for terminating the three month's old pregnancy in a fourteen-year-old girl who had been raped by five soldiers. The Oxford work would have been a landmark in the investigation of the foetus, and the results would have been accepted as the norm. The quality of the work was of the highest calibre, and the pictures are very valuable, but the conclusions reached were mainly wrong.

Many of the pictures show the radio-opaque material flowing down the superior vena cava to the right atrium. But there is one which shows the material flowing up the inferior vena cava. The article says, 'In the foetus, the inferior caval flow is composed of oxygenated blood returning to the heart from the placenta via the umbilical vein, *and venous blood from the lower segment.*' This is disgraceful, an assumption without any evidence to support it. The authors had gone to great lengths to investigate the foetal circulation, but not had the same quality of true scientific reasoning to support their claims. It then says, 'We have not as yet traced the course taken by this venous blood, our experiments having been confined to the demonstration of the flow from the umbilical vein.' It continues, 'The main portion of this stream, after entering the right auricle, passes through the foramen ovale to the left auricle and left ventricle.' This is another assumption. It is impossible to make out the details of the atria, and in any case, the picture they show is different from those that do show the right atrium, and therefore the injection would have most likely entered the left atrium, not the right. (The word 'auricle' is no longer used to describe an atrium). It seems to me that the authors were more intent on confirming the old wrong ideas rather than challenging them. At the beginning they say, 'the object of the foramen ovale is to allow re-oxygenated blood from the placenta to pass from the right auricle to the left side of the heart.' This is the fundamental error of the orthodox accounts. It is a pity they did not complete the investigation of the flow in the lower part of the inferior vena cava, it may have solved many of the problems, and revealed the true path of the venous return from the lower body to the right atrium. Instead, they may have been responsible for reassuring the authors of the modern medical works that they were correct and delayed the revelations of the secrets for generations.

In 1968, G. S. Dawes produced a book called, 'Foetal and Neonatal Physiology.' He also worked in Oxford and used the same method as the previous group. But his results were inferior to the others because he did not show any pictures, only his diagrams of his conclusions, which are quite bizarre and awfully wrong. As with the first group, he may have been responsible for concealing the truth of the foetal circulation for many years.

Now, I want to tell you about three main features of the orthodox accounts of the foetal circulation which are wrong.

1. The arterial blood from the placenta and the venous blood from the lower body in the inferior vena cava, entering the right atrium together separated by streaming.

    There is no doubt that some streaming in blood vessels does occur, but not of the respiratory gases in solution. Where there are different levels or pressures of oxygen and carbon-dioxide in solution close together, there is a rapid movement of each gas from higher to lower, resulting in equilibrium and a homogeneous mixture of both, with pressures midway between the two extremes. It is this extremely fast reaction which allows us to carry out the most strenuous of activities in the best of health. There was a good demonstration of it during the Oxford and Cambridge boat races on 7th April 2019. Some of the crews had sensors on their big toes which recorded their heart rates going up to more than 200 beats a minute. Their respiratory rates were also high, probably approaching the stroke rates of the oars at 40 breaths a minute. The flow of air in the lung airways, and the flow of blood in the capillaries of the lung respiratory zone would pass each other at excessive speeds, and in the briefest moment of time carbon-dioxide would pass from the lungs to the air, and oxygen would pass from the air into the blood. *Otherwise, all the crews would succumb from oxygen lack and excess carbon-dioxide. And if two separate streams of arterial and venous blood were to enter the foetal inferior vena cava side by side, the same reaction would lead immediately to a mixed homogeneous stream with low oxygen level and excess carbon-dioxide which would kill the foetus.* Separation of the respiratory gases by streaming cannot occur, it is a myth. Also, this arrangement would mean that all the three streams returning to the heart, the venous returns from the upper and lower bodies, and the placental stream, would enter the right atrium, with no stream entering the left atrium directly. This is preposterous.

2. How the arterial stream in the right atrium branches off from the venous stream to pass through the foramen ovale into the left atrium.

   The authors here are creating a new way of feeding the tissues without blood vessels, which is even worse than preposterous, it is crazy. D 6.

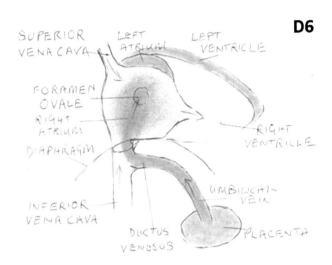

3. In the 1st edition of my book, I included a list of 18 of my books which accepted that the oxygenated blood from the placenta enters the right atrium and passes through the foramen ovale to the left atrium.

References
They are all taken from books that I have accumulated over the years, and that are still in my possession.
1. Gray's Anatomy 28th edn. 1942. Page 689.
2. Human Embryology and Morphology. 6th edn 1948 by Sir A. Keith. P453
3. A Textbook of Human Embryology 2nd. edn. 1963 by R.G. Harrison. P152
4. Cunningham's Textbook of Anatomy 10th edn 1964 P952
5. Developmental Anatomy 7th edn 1965 by L.B. Arey P392
6. Obstetric Anaesthesia 2nd edn 1965 by J. Selwyn Crawford P260
7. Samson Wright's Applied Physiology 11th edn. 1965 P502
8. Medical Physiology and Biochemistry 1968 by David Horrobin P418
9. Principles of Internal Medicine 6th edn 1970 Harrison p 1166
10. Anatomy 6th edn 1978 by R.J. Last P46
11. Human Embryology 1978 by M.J.T. Fitzgerald P175
12. Grant's Method of Anatomy 10th edn 1980 P33
13. Review of Medical Physiology 10th edn 1981 by W.F. Ganong P490
14. Textbook of Medical Physiology 6th edn 1981 by Guyton P1040
15. Basic Human Embryology 3rd edn 1984 by Smith and Williams P158
16. Human Physiology 1989 by Sheila Jennett P411
17. Langman's Medical Embryology 6th edn 1990 P221
18. Principles and Practice of Medicine 21st edn Davidson P629
All of the above works accept that the oxygenated blood from the placenta enters the right atrium and passes through the foramen ovale to the left atrium.

It seems logical enough, as the atria lie by side on each side of the septum. But is it true?

When two chambers of a heart are in series, each chamber contracts separately, in succession, first the atrium then the ventricle. Now the two atria do not beat in succession, they lie side by side and beat and relax together, and there cannot be a flow between them, either right to left or left to right, and all the orthodox accounts must be wrong.

Later in the year we flew home, and I introduced Pauline to my parents. We returned by sea, passing through the Mediterranean and Suez. Wherever we stopped, the purser, who was a tablemate, went ashore to search for the fruits Pauline craved for. She was pregnant, and our first offspring, Peter, was born in Salisbury, Rhodesia, on 31st March 1966.

A few weeks after we had returned from leave, on 11th November 1965, Noel Robertson, the Provincial Commissioner, invited us civil servants to meet in one of the hotels. At eleven o'clock we heard on the radio a strong emotional Ian Smith say, 'You have your Independence.' Noel asked us to stand and drink a toast to Rhodesia. This was the Unilateral Declaration of Independence, (U.D.I.) which no other country recognised. There were mixed feelings in the country, but those of us who stayed just knuckled down and got on with it.

At the end of May 1967, I was posted to Salisbury, and worked mainly in the large Harare hospital. My 5 years in the districts of rural Africa, the 3 years in the larger centres of Blantyre, Lilongwe and Zomba, and the 4-year trio in Fort Victoria of major surgery, general anaesthesia, and forensic medicine, came to an abrupt end, leaving behind the mortuary where the body of the little girl had uncovered the most precious secret of the foetal circulation.

The move to Salisbury proved to be a good one. Saturday morning clinical meetings were held there, and I gave four presentations, the first on 24th February 1968 concerned my findings in the foetal heart. In the audience was Hugh Philpott, the Rhodesian University professor of obstetrics and gynaecology. He introduced me to Professor A.P.D. Thompson, the dean and first professor of anatomy in the Rhodesian Medical School, who gave me the title of Honorary Research Officer and invited me to examine human foetuses in the anatomy department. I began by examining the foramen ovale and making drawings. I took the opportunity to visit the University Veterinary School library. I wanted to see if mammals other than the human had a foramen ovale. I thought they must have, but I wanted to confirm it. I read books on the anatomy of the horse, the dog, and the pig. Each one had a foramen ovale, but there was another feature common to all of them and ourselves. I wondered why those 'lower' creatures should have what we have in our anatomy, was it important? I then realised its true function in us all. It was '*The Azygos Vein*', which connects the two venae cavae. Its lower end arises from the back of the inferior vena cava, (IVC), at the level of the renal veins, branches off the IVC and passes

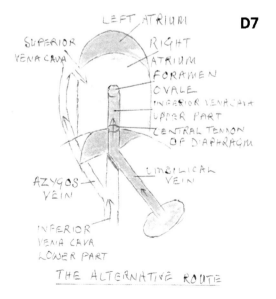

35

up through the diaphragm, arches forwards over the root of the right lung and joins the superior vena cava. *So, in the foetus, there is an alternative route for the venous return from the lower body to reach the right atrium,* and there must be an obstruction, or block, in the inferior vena cava above the diversion to prevent the lower return from mixing with the placental return. Also, note that in the foetus the right atrium has only one vena cava, the superior, and both the upper and lower venous returns pass through it to enter the atrium. See my diagram D 7. Later, I realised that the inferior vena cava must be divided functionally into upper and lower parts, the upper to carry the placental stream into the left atrium, and the lower to carry the lower venous return into the right atrium. (I have never actually seen the azygos vein; I probably removed it when I cut off each foetal head. But there must be an azygos vein, the foetus cannot live without it).

Without doubt, the azygos vein was the third secret to be uncovered, the block would be the fourth, and the solitary superior vena cava the fifth.

I reflected on my twelve years in the government medical service and felt competent to manage a wide variety of medical and surgical conditions, but there was something which bothered me, Psychiatry. I knew so little about it, especially of those cases of mania I had seen. Then, out of the blue, towards the end of 1968, I was asked to take over the running of the newly opened Psychiatric Unit in the grounds of Harare hospital. It was to be a temporary measure until a psychiatrist could be appointed. But as the weeks and months went by without one, I continued in charge, and began to explore the subject myself, helped by the friendly senior psychiatric nurse, Mr. C. Kinsey from Nottingham, who eased me gently into it. I was beginning to understand the subject more and more, and realised it was fundamentally no different from the other branches of medicine, which depended on my five pillars of wisdom: a sound knowledge of anatomy, physiology, and pathology, a good history, and an adequate examination. (cf. T.E. Lawrence of Arabia).

On my first day there I witnessed a patient being given straight ECT. (electro-convulsive therapy without sedation). It distressed me. Two nurses stood on each side of the conscious patient, ready to hold the four limbs during the convulsion. Mr Kinsey held the head, with a gag in the patient's mouth to prevent the tongue from being bitten. Then he switched on the machine which was connected to the patient's head by a wet electrode on each temple. There followed a massive convulsion, with limbs stiffened and clenching of the teeth, followed by muscular spasms and salivation. The patient slowly regained consciousness and was returned to the ward. Another patient suffered back pain, which was probably due to a compressed fracture of a thoracic vertebra. I stopped all this and asked for a Boyle's machine for the Unit. My experience of muscle relaxants in Fort Victoria proved useful, and I wanted to introduce them in the Unit without pentothal and with the patient fully conscious. This drug, being an anti-convulsant, means giving more ECT than was necessary, and the patient would take a long time to wake up and be watched by the staff. But the muscle fibrillations which followed the giving of scoline were believed to be painful. I experimented and asked for one of the staff to be paralysed by the scoline, fully conscious while I respirated him, the volunteer to be given a day off work. Jeremiah came forward, and I paralysed and respirated him with oxygen for about five minutes until he could breathe on his own. *The fibrillations had caused no pain.* From that time onwards, no straight ECT was given, and my own method was used for every patient needing convulsive therapy. No pain, no gag, no staff at each side, no salivation, no fractures, no intubation, just the mask held over the mouth while I pumped the balloon, and with just the slightest twitching of his face to show he was having a convulsion. We never had any complication from that day, and each patient was sent back to the ward fully conscious. I believe it is the convulsion, not the shock, which is beneficial.

I described these things in my annual report for 1968, and my annual report for 1969 was 13 pages long, giving a comprehensive account of the Unit and our work there. It included the diagnosis, treatment, and result of each of the 790 patients we admitted. The Harare Hospital Medical Superintendent's secretary baulked at having to include the list of patients, and he allowed her to omit it, which was a pity because it contained so much valuable clinical material and the results of our treatment.

It became clear, as I spent more days in the Unit, that those men I had seen in Nyasaland and those whom we admitted to the Unit with mania, had been drinking alcohol in excess, and as I began to understand the cause, I modified the treatment, giving less ECT towards the end of my stay there, compared to the many times it had been given initially. I drew this graph which summarises the management of these cases. I believe, without treatment they would slowly get better and for a short time be normal, followed by a period of depression and eventually return to normality. Giving the modern anti-psychotic drugs would result in a similar pattern but shorter in time, and giving ECT would make the recovery to normality even quicker. These things were also included in my report for 1969.

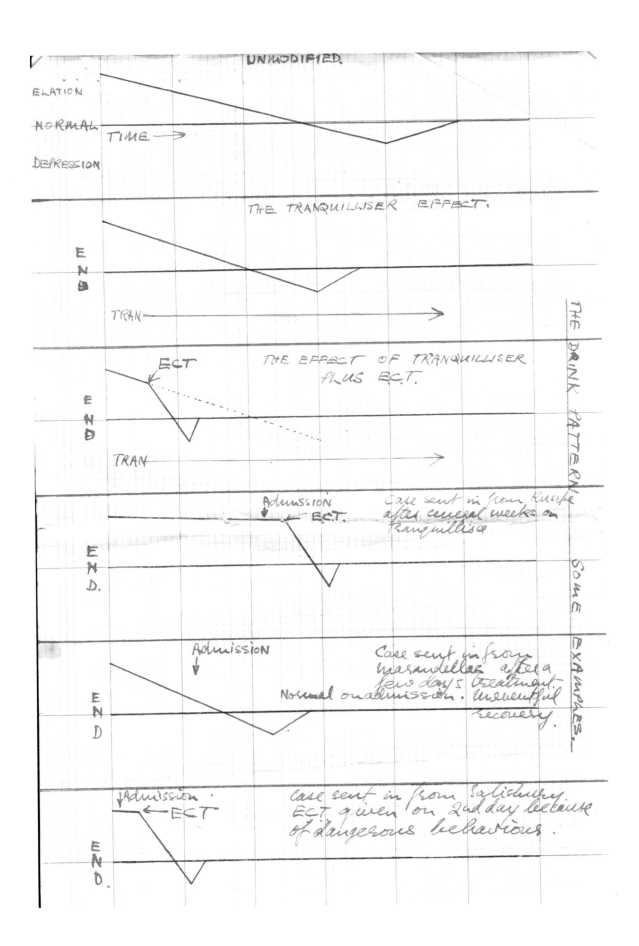

UNMODIFIED.

ELATION

NORMAL   TIME →

DEPRESSION

THE TRANQUILLISER EFFECT.

E
N
D

TRAN →

ECT   THE EFFECT OF TRANQUILLISER
        PLUS E.C.T.

E
N
D

TRAN →

Admission   Case sent in from Rusape
     ←E.C.T.   after several weeks on
              tranquilliser

E
N
D.

Admission   Case sent in from
             marandellas after a
             few days treatment.
Normal on admission. Uneventful
              recovery.

E
N
D

Admission   Case sent in from Salisbury
  ←ECT   ECT given on 2nd day because
             of dangerous behaviour.

E
N
D.

THE DRINK PATTERN. SOME EXAMPLES.

38

Some years later, when I was in general practice, two UNESCO psychiatrists from Galway in Ireland, visited Harare. The senior one was Brian Leonard, the professor of pharmacology there, who impressed me. They gave lectures on psychiatry to the government doctors and to the G.P.'s who wished to come, such as myself. These were very helpful, and I was able to understand them because the professor was lucid and clever in his delivery, but also because there was agreement between what he said and what I had learned in the Psychiatric Unit. Psychiatry is all about pharmacology, or much of its treatment as I had learned in the Unit. They visited us twice more, and on the last one visited the Unit, accompanied by many of us. I asked the professor if he would like to see my annual report, and he took it to read. The next day he returned it and said it should be published. I have not done so, but perhaps there is still time. Even later, I met Mr. and Mrs. Kinsey when I was visiting a patient in a home for the elderly they had opened. Spontaneously, at the same time as we hugged each other, I said, 'I learned a lot from you,' and he said, 'you taught me a lot.'

Since seeing the features of the little 'girl' who had died without breathing, I understood that it is the *foetus,* which is delivered, and that the foetus changes into a baby after the delivery when the first deep breath is taken. This was a remarkable revelation of the relation of the foetus to the baby, which can now be called the *sixth secret of the foetal circulation,* and I was very interested in a television programme which showed the birth of a foal, and I followed it carefully. At first, the non-breathing, lifeless-looking animal with a narrow unexpanded chest, was delivered on to the ground. Then, almost immediately, it took a deep breath, opened its chest, stood up on all four legs and shook itself. My belief was confirmed, I had seen a foetus change into a foal. In another programme on television, I watched the delivery of a goat kid. It emerged in a flaccid lifeless form and did not breathe. It was stillborn, and I knew I had watched the delivery of a foetus. I then realised that stillborn farm animals could be a valuable source of information on the foetal circulation if human foetuses were unavailable.

At the end of 1969 I resigned from the government medical service, and in April the following year opened my own medical practice in the pleasant Harare suburb of Greendale, leaving the university work and putting off further investigation of the foetus until another day. This came much later than I had expected, and in 2004, when I had become an octogenarian, it began to occupy my mind more and more. When I qualified, I had become a Bachelor, of medicine and surgery. But after marriage, and Pauline having given us four children, I thought Doctor would be more appropriate. I tried to submit my work for an MD, but previous and private work was no longer acceptable. I therefore decided to do, what I had never considered before, to produce my own little book. It was published in Zimbabwe in 2011, rather amateurish, but it was a start, and if I had not begun then I might not have reached the present position, where I have been able to explore and develop my ideas further. In February 2013, Pauline had to have an operation. The surgery was successful, but she developed acute pancreatitis, probably from the anaesthetic, and died in intensive care three weeks later. I returned to England in the following June, having lived in Africa for 59 years, to live with my son Andrew and his wife Kim and family, in Oswestry, where I have continued to write new versions of my book. In Zimbabwe, I had not handled a mobile phone or a laptop, and in my nineties, I had to learn both, Kim helping me to jump from typewriter to computer, and together with Andrew, providing those home comforts which made my precipitate arrival in Oswestry such a pleasant one.

Why we did not have a cold room in the mortuary.

When I had my own practice, one of my patients had been a policeman in Fort Victoria and had had to attend the post-mortems he was involved with. *He told me the doctors did not do the post-mortems,* they were done by the old ambulance driver, who also supervised the cleaning of the hospital. So that was the answer, no need to give him a cold room, the medical superintendent or his junior never went near the mortuary and must have made up the cause of death from the result given by the ambulance driver. This was disgraceful and may had led to wrongful sentences of murder for the defendants. But perhaps the old man may have become quite good at working out the causes of death. These things would have happened after I had left Fort Vic and may have happened before I had arrived. Rhodesia, as it was then called after the break-up of the Federation, was going through a difficult time, and many of us whites were leaving the country, reducing the number of doctors available.

The best of my thoughts on my work on the foetus come in the night, and I must get up and record them in my computer, otherwise I might lose them. Sometimes, they are better than before, and I have to publish another version. But sometimes I remember some of the best work which had gone before, and it would be included in the current one. This happened with the fifth edition, published in 2018, some parts of which are notable because it was the first one to include pictures of my work on foetal lambs taken with my mobile phone, and I have reproduced one of them here, on the right, unnumbered. It had been given to me by Graham

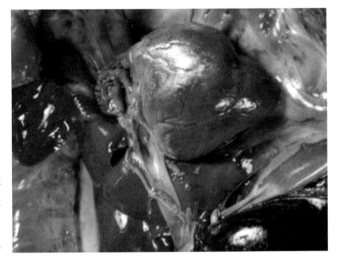

Jones, a sheep farmer near Oswestry on the border with Wales. For the second time since 1965, I had been able to see the inferior vena cava leading to the foramen ovale, this one in a foetal lamb, the other in a human foetus.

The findings in the little 'girl's body in April 1965, and this picture from the 5th edition, were of the greatest value in helping me to understand the foetal circulation, they lay the foundation of the plan, which I have shown in diagram D 8. The arterial blood from the left atrium enters the left ventricle and is carried in the aorta to the junction with pulmonary trunk, the end of which is called the ductus arteriosus. The blood supply for the upper body comes off the upper aorta, and the venous return enters the right atrium through the

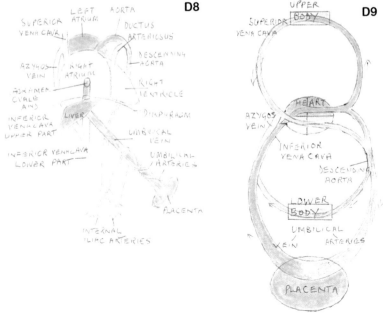

superior vena cava. Beyond the junction the descending aorta carries a mixture of arterial and venous blood to the lower body and to the placenta by the two umbilical arteries. This diagram shows how the arterial return from the placenta enters the left atrium through the umbilical vein, the inferior vena cava and the foramen ovale, and how the venous return from the lower body enters the right atrium through the azygos vein and the superior vena cava. In this other diagram, D 9, I have separated the umbilical arteries from the umbilical vein on either side of the placenta. It gives a simpler plan which is easier to follow.

We can now go round the plan and discuss each part.

The Junction.

It is a remarkable feature, where two different streams meet and flow in the same vessel, combined into one stream of mixed blood for the lower body and placenta. In the realms of anatomy and physiology it is entirely new to us. It has been misunderstood and could not have been seen by some of those who have described it. It is often shown wrongly with the ductus arteriosus leading into the side of the aorta. It does not enter the aorta, it lies at the side of the aorta and the two vessels lying side by side with a narrow angle between them, converge together to form the beginning of the descending aorta, as I had seen when I examined that specimen in my home. Both vessels are derivatives of the paired primitive arterial arches, the aorta from the 4th arches and the ductus from the 6th arches. The 5th arches are said to have disappeared without trace, but I suspect that they had developed into the two coronary arteries. Arising from the aortic arch in the human are three large vessels, the brachiocephalic trunk, the left common carotid artery, and the left subclavian artery. It is important to note that the ductus, carrying venous blood, joins the arch beyond the left subclavian artery, preventing contamination of the arterial supply for the upper body and ensuring a rich supply of arterial blood for the brain. In the lamb, only one large vessel arises from the aortic arch. I have called it the cephalic artery. An earlier group from Oxford had called it brachiocephalic, which is more appropriate because it supplies the upper limbs as well as the head.

The circulation for the upper body.

The upper body of the foetus is richly supplied with arterial blood from the aorta proximal to the junction. It is the most important part of the circulation for the foetus, which supplies many parts, and which shows the importance of them in the assembly of the new creature. They include the heart, the brain, the breasts, the eyes ears nose and mouth, the thyroid and thymus, and the upper limbs. The venous return drains into the right atrium through the superior vena cava, except for the return from the heart, which drains directly into the coronary sinus of the heart before entering the right atrium. See diagram D 10.

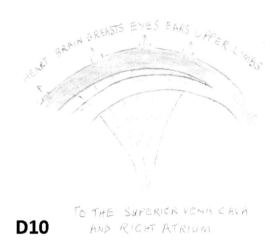

D10

The circulation for the lower body.

The lower body includes those structures below the diaphragm, which are fed with mixed blood from the descending aorta. They are the abdominal viscera, the genital organs, the lower limbs and much of the

41

chest wall. The venous return from the lower body flows through the lower part of the inferior vena cava, through the azygos vein and superior vena cava to the right atrium, as I have shown you before. Because of the difference between the quality of the blood for the upper and lower parts of the circulation, the two parts would be segregated, *and we can now call the segregation the 7ʰ secret.*

I see this segregation as part of the design which would reduce the size of the lower body, giving preference to the development of the upper body. The gestation period is reduced, the brain is allowed to mature quicker to take on its numerous future responsibilities, the head is better shaped and better prepared for the delivery obstetrics, and the hands will be needed early to respond to the orders from the brain, while the abdominal viscera, the genital organs and the legs will be able to develop later after birth.

The circulation for the placenta.

The placenta is also fed with mixed blood from the descending aorta, and branching off the internal iliac arteries are the two umbilical arteries, which ascend on the anterior abdominal wall to the umbilicus and travel outside the foetus to the placenta on the uterine wall. See my diagram D 11. The placenta is in two parts, a foetal part which receives the umbilical arteries, and a maternal part supplied by the uterine arteries, with the interface between them, across which the respiratory gases, food, and waste pass in solution. The meeting of the two takes place in little lakes or lacunae embedded in the uterine wall, which are supplied with blood flowing through them from the uterine arteries to the uterine veins. The venous portion of the mixed blood passing through the placenta from the foetal to the maternal part, enters the lacunae in little chorionic vascular tufts or villi, and it is the capillaries of the villi, washed by maternal blood, which are the interface. Diagram D 12. The umbilical arteries, travelling through the amniotic fluid, having no external blood supply, would depend on the oxygen of the mixed stream passing through them, either directly through the endothelial lining or from the vasa vasorum, while the foetal side of the placenta would also depend on the oxygen of the mixed stream coming from the foetal left ventricle, and as the oxygen passes through the umbilical arteries and placenta, it would be used up in producing the energy for the metabolism of those parts and replaced by carbon-dioxide. The venous portion of

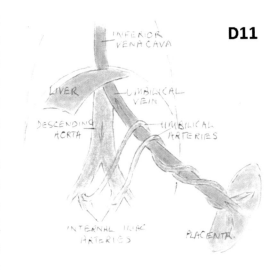

D11

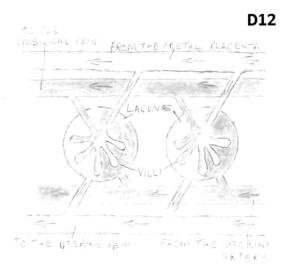

D12

the mixed stream coming from the foetal right ventricle and sent to the placenta to be changed into arterial for the foetus, is then added to the carbon-dioxide produced in the placenta, and all the blood reaching the interface would be venous. The maternal side would then receive the carbon-dioxide and waste, and give in return to the umbilical vein, oxygen and food for the umbilical vein and the foetus, and oxygen and food for the umbilical arteries and the placenta. (Yes, the placenta needs oxygen and food too). The arterial replenished blood returning from the placenta in the umbilical vein flows to the liver. I think some would feed the liver and be changed into the correct food for the foetus and placenta, which is then discharged through the hepatic veins into the upper part of the inferior vena cava. The rest would pass through the ductus venosus and flow together with the flow from the liver through the central tendon of the diaphragm to the foramen ovale and the left atrium. The mixed blood supply for the placenta would be larger than the mixed blood supply for the lower body because the arterial blood produced by the placenta must supply both parts of the foetus and the placenta as well.

The circulation for the lungs.

In many of the books on the foetus, the lungs are mentioned without a mention of an arterial blood supply. They may be sidelined off the main stream without a function and unopened, (not collapsed, collapse is a pathological condition affecting the lungs after they have already opened), but they are so important and must be well fed and supplied with oxygen to keep them in tip-top condition for the moment of birth, when with the heart they will play the key role of keeping the body alive.

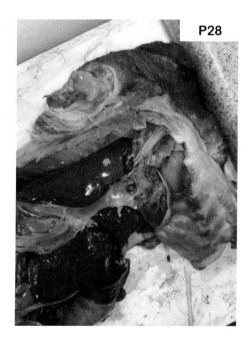

P28

In the lambing season of 2019, I examined a foetal lamb which showed a channel branching off the inferior vena cava close to the foramen ovale, and I took this picture with my mobile phone camera. P 28. The channel is shown leading into the right atrium above the opening of the coronary sinus. Between the ends of the channel and the coronary sinus is a crescentic blade which probably converts the end of each vessel into a valve preventing backflow in atrial systole. This unnamed channel is very important, providing oxygen and food for the right atrium where it mixes with the venous blood from the superior vena cava carrying carbon-dioxide and waste. Most of this mixed blood would be carried to the right ventricle, the pulmonary trunk, the ductus arteriosus and the descending aorta, *but some would enter the pulmonary arteries and feed the lungs.* It is an unusual arrangement with the pulmonary arteries carrying oxygen and food to the lungs and returning to the left atrium with carbon-dioxide and waste.

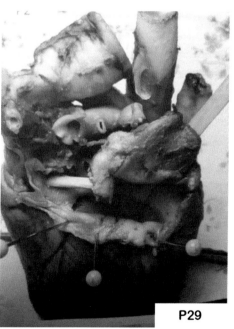

A year earlier I had taken this other picture in the 5th edition, without realising its importance. It shows a long stick in the superior vena cava and a short stick propping up the inferior vena cava which I have cut open, revealing the foramen ovale at the far end, and the unnamed vessel leading into the right atrium above the opening of the coronary sinus. Such a valuable picture,

P29

giving clearly the anatomical details of this part of the heart which feeds the foetal lungs. *The eighth precious secret.*

I invite you to stay a while and consider the features of this second picture. Included is an excellent view of that branch of the inferior vena cava which feeds the lungs, *and which had never been shown before.* Of all the standard books of anatomy physiology and medicine which I possess, not one has a photograph on any part of the foetal circulation, and the accounts they give of the circulation and birth changes are all wrong. What we need are facts, accurate observations, supported by photographs or drawings if possible. We can see the features, superficial and deep of this picture because of the remarkable quality of the lenses in the modern mobile phones. I don't think they had arrived in 1965, and I did try to capture the features of the little heart I had taken from the mortuary by drawing them accurately. When my drawings disappeared, I had nothing to support my plan of the foetal circulation but a few sketches, but picture P 29 more than compensates for the loss. It gives an excellent view of the coronary sinus leading into the right atrium, above it the unnamed vessel which feeds the lungs, and a remarkable inside view of the inferior vena cava leading to the foramen ovale at the far end. In the first version of my book, I said that the mouth of the inferior vena cava was closely and accurately applied round the foramen ovale. Now we can see in picture P 29 how closely and accurately the mouth of the inferior vena cava is applied round the foramen ovale. Where else do we see the inside of a blood vessel? Picture P 29 is so rare and beautiful, it stands alone as the best photograph ever taken of two newly discovered pieces of anatomy, the inferior vena cava leading directly to the foramen ovale, and the unnamed branch of inferior vena cava feeding the lungs. *More than that, it is the climax of all my many years' work on the foetal circulation.*

Now, I want to show you a little drawing I made on the 18th of April 1965, when I had first begun to explore the foetus, even before finding the truth in the little 'girl' in the mortuary. It shows the mouths of the pulmonary arteries inside the pulmonary trunk of a small premature one-day old human foetus delivered in Fort Victoria hospital at the end of March 1965. The mouths are side by side and so positioned as to indicate that they had been intentionally designed to capture the flow from the pulmonary trunk. Interesting, isn't it, at each end we see a special arrangement; at the beginning we see the origin of the arterial stream from the inferior vena cava, and at the end we see the special design of the pulmonary trunk for catching the mixed stream for the lungs.

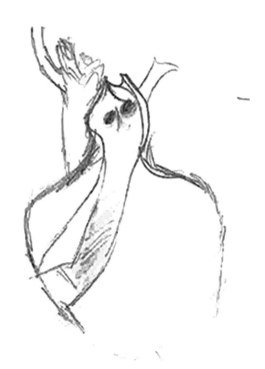

Though the lungs would be non-functional, each cell would be carefully attended to and prepared for the day of birth when it will immediately become responsible for the respiratory exchanges. The lungs therefore would be very vascular and large. If you will return to picture P 28, you will see that though I have removed part of the right lung to expose the channel feeding the lungs, the lungs occupy a large part of the chest and would cover the heart. In diagram D 13, I have tried to show the anatomy of the chest organs, the lower body, and the placenta, and I have shown the large size of the lungs by the faintly drawn criss-cross lines. I have omitted the captions, which would spoil it, and by now I hope you will understand the details of the foetal circulation.

D13

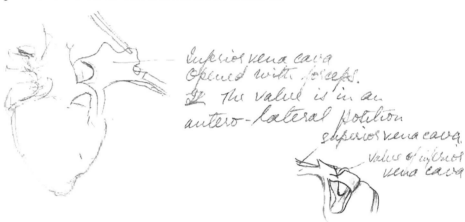

I have more to say about picture 29. The unnamed vessel branching off the inferior vena cava, (IVC), is none-other than what has been wrongly called the valve of the IVC. There is no such thing as the valve of the IVC, the people who describe it have never seen it, and can have only imagined it. Some books say wrongly that it helps to direct arterial blood from the IVC into the left atrium, and some call it the Eustachian valve. There are no photographs of it, only diagrams. In the same drawing I showed you of the mouths of the pulmonary arteries, there is another which shows the upper part of the IVC close to the foetal heart. I had called it the valve of the IVC, but I had been misled, the only possible feature on the upper part of the IVC close to the heart would be the channel I had found leading to the right atrium. I had taken a picture of the channel in 2018 and drawn it in 1965. Such a precious drawing, the only one ever made of the channel, wrongly called the valve of the inferior vena cava.

The lambing season occurs once a year in March and April, and if I miss collecting a specimen, I must wait a year before I can collect another. This year, I was only able to collect one stillborn lamb, and it had some unusual congenital features, and I will have to wait until next year before I can collect another. In June 2022, I had a stroke, which affected my speech and my right hand, and made my balance problems even worse. My daughter Mary and her husband Bernard invited me to leave my flat in Oswestry and move down to live with them and their family in Horley, Surrey. I gladly accepted, and moved down in the following September, leaving behind Andrew and Kim, and sheep farmer Graham Jones, my source of supply for stillborn lambs, and in the spring of 2023, I again had no specimen to examine.

Because of my stroke I have been more cautious than normal in checking my work, and I was disappointed to find that I had made a mistake in several of my diagrams; the aorta does not rise up behind the left atrium, it rises up in front of it. I tried to copy the diagrams which showed the error, and draw the correct

arrangement, but my trembling right hand made it very difficult, and the results were not good. I therefore decided to leave the diagrams as they were and change the text which accompanied them. The first diagram with the error is D 14, on this page, and I have changed the text to 'Rising up in front of the left atrium is the aorta' in the next paragraph of this page. Diagrams D20 and D 21 are on page 51, D22 is on page 53, and D 23 is on page 56.

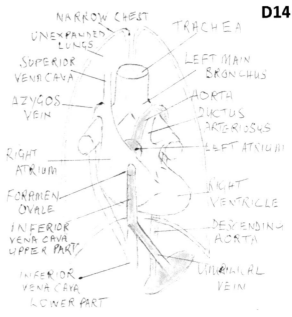

D14

The butcher supplied me with a lamb's heart connected to the lungs and liver as I had asked, which allowed me to refresh my memory of the lamb's anatomy, and see those parts involved in the change from foetal. These are, the branching of the pulmonary trunk into two, with no ductus arteriosus joining the aorta, the large, inflated lungs instead of the smaller unexpanded foetal ones, the fossa ovalis replacing the foramen ovale, and both venae cavae supplying the right atrium instead of the azygos vein and the superior vena cava. The human heart has four pulmonary veins leading to the left atrium, in the lamb there are only two, one from each lung. Making use of the features of a lamb's heart, and using diagram D 8 as a guide, I then made diagram, D 14, showing the foetal features as I imagined them to be. Posteriorly, is the buff-coloured trachea branching into the two main bronchi. Centrally placed between the two main bronchi is the upper part of the left atrium. Rising up in front of the left atrium is the aorta, which curves over the left main bronchus in company with the ductus arteriosus. To the right of the left atrium is the superior vena cava, with the azygos vein rolling over the right main bronchus to join it. The superior vena cava leads into the right atrium below and in front of the left atrium, and the right atrium leads into the right ventricle. The short left pulmonary artery is shown coming off the

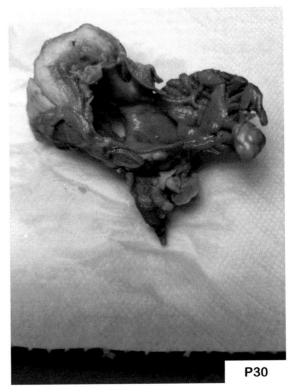

P30

pulmonary trunk and feeding the left lung, but the longer right pulmonary artery is not visible, it passes behind the superior vena cava to reach the right lung. The aorta and the ductus arteriosus meet to form the descending aorta which descends behind the heart carrying mixed blood to the lower body and the placenta. Fresh arterial blood leaves the placenta in the umbilical vein and is carried to the inferior vena cava which leads it through the central tendon of the diaphragm, and through the right atrium to the foramen ovale and the left atrium. On each side are the un-expanded lungs. I will have to check these things if and when the next stillborn lamb arrives.

Departing from imagination, and coming back to reality with this same specimen supplied by the butcher, I was unable to include the two pulmonary veins returning from the lungs to the left atrium, but I did carefully examine the interior of the left atrium and the entrances of the veins, and I took this picture, P 30, on 10th December 2021, of that part of the left atrium containing them, which I had removed and

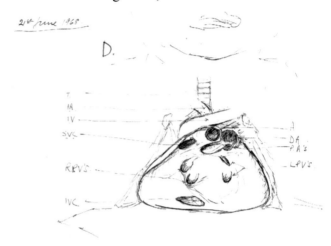

preserved in 10% formalin. I was particularly interested in the pulmonary veins and the way they entered the left atrium because in one of my drawings of the human foetus which I had made in the medical school in 1968, drawing D seen on the right, the entrances, (RPV's and LPV's) appeared to be valvular. Of the three good books of anatomy that I possess, one of them does not mention valves for the pulmonary veins, and the other two deny that the pulmonary veins have valves. In picture P 30, the openings of the two pulmonary veins are seen close to the upper border of the left atrium. Between them is a rounded ridge, with the right opening at the end of a tunnel and the left emerging under part of the atrial wall. *These are without doubt, valves.* They may not look like valves, having no cusps or chordae tendineae, but they are valves, nevertheless. During atrial contraction the roof of each tunnel would have been held tightly against the floor, closing the tunnels, and preventing backflow. These valves deserve names. They cannot be called pulmonary because it is the name of the exit from the right ventricle. 'Tunnel' is more appropriate,' the tunnel valves of the left atrium,' passing through the atrial wall, two in the lamb, and four in the human.

The pumps in our bodies have two components, muscles which do the work and valves which give direction to the blood flows. Each pump has two valves, inlet, and outlet. I believe that inlet valves are opened actively by the muscles attached to them, while outlet valves are opened passively by the weight of the blood pushing the cusps aside. All the pumping chambers of the heart have inlet and outlet valves, but they are not of the same design, different functions, different designs. The right atrium may not seem to have an inlet valve, but the musculi pectinati are so arranged that with each beat from the pacemaker they cause a wave of contraction to pass down the atrium and milk the blood into the right ventricle, acting like a valve to prevent backflow. *Prevention of backflow,* that is the criterion which tells us there is a valve. In the postnate, backflow to the lungs is prevented by the tunnel valves in the left atrium, there can be no circulation, no life without them. In the human foetus, there are five valves in the left atrium, the foramen ovale in the anterior wall of the atrium preventing backflow into the inferior vena cava, and the four smaller tunnel valves in the posterior wall preventing backflow into the pulmonary veins and lungs. In the foetal lamb there are two small tunnel valves in the left atrium, and we can now claim the tunnel valves to be *the ninth hidden secret.* Can we not also claim picture 30 to be another one of the best photographs ever taken of a newly discovered piece of anatomy?

We have been taught that the heart contracts in systole and relaxes in diastole. This is wrong, it also works in diastole. In my discussions on valves in the previous editions of my book, I showed how my own atrial fibrillation, (A.F.), helped me to understand how cardiac muscle does not relax in diastole. The atrioventricular valves are mixed, outlet for the atria and inlet for the ventricles. In A.F., the ventricles get little or no help from the malfunctioning atria and do most or all the work in both diastole and systole. The atrioventricular, A-V, valves then become pure inlet valves, opening actively in ventricular diastole, and closing actively in ventricular systole. Every person, including myself, walking around with A.F., is living proof of the ventricles working in diastole, we cannot live without them. There must be two sets of cardiac muscle, close together, one to open the a-v valves and the ventricles while the other relaxes, and another to close them when the first relaxes. I have not heard of A.F. affecting one atrium, and I presume the fault may lie in the pacemaker, rather than in the atria.

Returning to the left atrium and its cardiac muscle wall, in the postnate, one set of muscle would open the tunnels in diastole, allowing fresh blood from the lungs to enter, and the other set would close them in systole, preventing backflow to the lungs and ejecting the blood into the left ventricle through the mitral valve.

It is not always made clear what the electrocardiogram, (ECG), represents. It certainly does not represent the cardiac impulse generated by the pacemaker in the right atrium. The cardiac impulse is but a fuse which ignites every movable part of the heart packed with high explosive, *and it is the movement of each part of the heart which generates the electricity, the pattern of which is recorded by the ECG.* After each movement, the high explosive is replenished with food and oxygen from the coronary circulation. Let us look at the ECG.

As the blood is pumped by the heart from one part to the next, each movement is revealed by the ECG. There is also a relation to the heart sounds, *which can only be heard when the ventricles close.* The filling and emptying of the atria is a slow process, as we can see from the long P wave on the ECG. The upward R wave represents the opening of the a-v valves and the ventricles, while the longer and stronger downward S wave represents the closing of the a-v valves and the ventricles, which cause the 'LUB' of the first heart sound as the ventricles eject their blood into the aorta and pulmonary trunk.

The outlets of the aorta and the pulmonary trunk are each guarded by tricuspid valves, 120 degrees wide at the base of each cusp, and each cusp ending in a thickened point above, with the sides free from their neighbours, and when the ventricles eject their blood, it rebounds from the aorta and pulmonary trunk, causing high pressure *retrograde* waves, which snap close both valves and ventricles, making the louder 'DUP' of the second heart sound. The 'T' wave of the ECG is probably caused by the rebounding *walls* of the aorta and pulmonary trunk.

The wall of the aorta, but not of the pulmonary trunk, bulges outwards opposite each cusp, making an aortic sinus, and leading off from the anterior sinus is the right coronary artery, while from the left posterior sinus the left coronary artery begins, and with each heartbeat the heart is fed by both coronary arteries with arterial blood.

To the right of this description, you will see the ECG displayed, with the letters LUB and DUP above.

We can go a little deeper into the valve mechanism. The foramen ovale has two septa, primum and secundum. In atrial diastole they are separated by the muscles attached to them and there is a pressure difference between low outside and negative inside, and blood flows into the left atrium. In atrial systole the pressure inside the atrium is greatly increased by the strength of the atrial muscles, which close the atrium and close the septa together and force the blood past the mitral valve into the left ventricle.

I can now show you some of the pictures I took when I was examining the entrances of the pulmonary veins inside the left atrium of the lamb's heart.

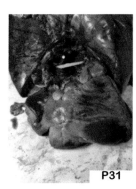
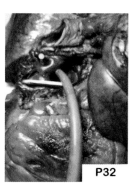
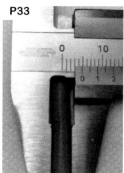
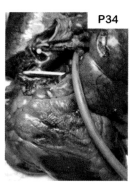

In the first, P 31, the left atrium is held open by a stick and some pins, with the entrance of the left vein above the stick, and the entrance of the right vein below the stick. The second picture, P 32, shows a soft rubber catheter, which I have inserted into the right pulmonary vein. P 33 shows the catheter, almost 5 mm in diameter in the blades of my mini calliper, while in the last picture, P 34, I have inserted the catheter into the left pulmonary vein. These valuable pictures allow the readers to judge for themselves, whether they agree with me or not that these tunnels are valves.

The Foetal Heart Sounds.

The two sounds made by the postnatal heart measure the duration of ventricular systole, with the softer 'lub' heard as the ventricles contract and close the atrioventricular valves, and the harsher 'dup' occurring when the ventricles begin to open and the outlet valves close. The left ventricular sounds are louder than the right sounds and we need only to consider them. The a-v valve is the mitral and the outlet is the aortic. In the foetus there is an extra sound made by the closing of the foramen ovale in atrial systole. It is much softer than the other two and more difficult to hear, because atrial muscle is much weaker than ventricular muscle, and when the left atrium contracts in systole the closing valve causes little vibration in the valve and the surrounding blood. But it can be heard nevertheless, and it occurs just before the other two as the atrium contracts immediately before the onset of ventricular systole. There will therefore be a triple gallop rhythm; soft lub, louder lub and harsher dup. Diagram D 15. Anyone with a Doppler foetal heart monitor should be able find this gallop rhythm in the later months of pregnancy. Move the machine about and you will find the difference between the slower double rhythm from the mother's heart, and the

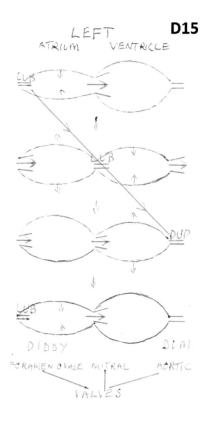

faster gallop rhythm heard elsewhere; diddy-dum, diddy-dum, diddy-dum. With the left atrium being a posterior chamber, the triple rhythm would be more easily heard from the back of the foetus. Also, the flexed position of the foetus would keep the front of the chest away from the probing monitor.

In the postnate, the two sounds tell us about the ventricles, how they measure the length of ventricular systole. In the foetus, the triple rhythm tells us about the left atrium, how it is pumping blood into the left ventricle from the inferior vena cava. *We have uncovered the tenth hidden secret.*

In 2017, when I was investigating the heart sounds, I scanned the lower abdomens of the young ladies in the supermarket without finding a likely subject, but outside waiting for a bus was a young girl with a large abdomen. I asked her if I could listen to the foetal heart, but she wasn't pregnant, just fat. She was very polite and did not give me a slap. I then went to the pharmacy where one of the assistants looked a possible candidate. She wasn't pregnant but pointed to the assistant at the perfumes counter whom she knew to be pregnant. I went along to her, and she readily agreed to help. On 19th November 2017, I took a taxi to her home and listened to her foetal heart with my Doppler, with her husband watching nearby. On the right side of her abdomen, I could only hear the double rhythm, but on the left side I picked up the gallop quickly, even without my hearing aid, and she and her husband heard it too. I did not examine her otherwise and did not give her any medical advice, I only explained why there should be the triple rhythm I was searching for. So, my visit on that Sunday morning to a lady who was not a patient of mine, and in the cause of medical science, was not unethical. I was so grateful to her, and so excited. I bubbled over in the taxi going home. Later, she showed me a picture of her new-born baby. What a strong handsome fellow. No wonder we all heard his triple rhythm so easily.

The Birth Changes.

A bright new light which illuminated the long-hidden secrets of the foetal circulation in April 1965, had been switched on by the death of the little girl who had failed to breathe after her delivery. Why she did not breathe we will never know, but we will know that the normal transition from foetus to baby is due to the onset of breathing. The light is never switched on again and we are kept in the dark during the transition. We can see the waking the breathing and the crying, but the internal changes are shielded from us and have never been seen. But if we have been able to recognise correctly how the foetus differs from the baby, we will be more able to work out/guess the hidden changes which must occur at birth. As they depend on breathing, they cannot occur in the mother, they take place outside the mother after the delivery. The creature which is delivered is therefore a foetus, and the birth of the baby takes place after the delivery when the first deep breath is taken. The little 'girl' who had died in 1965 would also have been a foetus, and it was her foetal features which had shone so brightly on that April day.

In a previous edition of my book, I described the changes in two parts, both occurring outside the mother, the dismantling of the placental circulation when the foetus is delivered, and the changes which follow the delivery when

D16

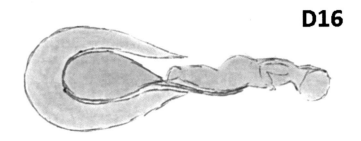

the foetus takes the first deep breath. I now believe the two parts function together. Let me show you the first part.

When the delivery is completed and the foetus leaves the mother, the emptied contracted uterus will squash the placenta and stop the circulation within it and within all the vessels of the cord, and the foetus will be denied a blood supply. See D 16. There will be a double effect, with the stopping of the flow in the umbilical vein to the foetus, and the stopping of the flow in the umbilical arteries to the placenta. Usually, there would be a continuous flow of oxygenated blood in the umbilical vein for the foetus as the uterus mangles the placenta and wrings out the blood, but the flow will eventually cease when the placenta has been exsanguinated. The effect on the placenta will be more dramatic; there may be pulsation in the umbilical arteries but there can be no flow into the squashed placenta, and the large cardiac output of mixed blood for the placenta will be diverted to the lower body of the foetus and changed into venous for the right atrium. The foetus will therefore gain from oxygenated blood for the left atrium and venous blood for the right atrium and will be well cared for naturally at this time when the placental circulation is dismantled.

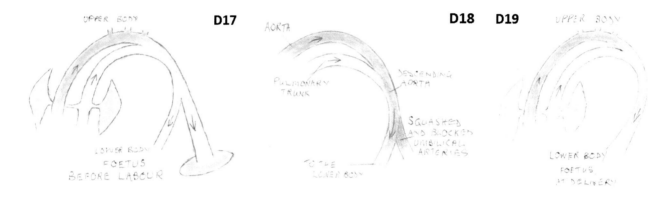

There are three diagrams here. D 17 shows the position before labour with the placenta receiving the larger share of mixed blood. D 18 shows how the mixed blood is diverted from the placenta to the lower body during the delivery, and D 19, again at the delivery without the placenta. The tissues fed by the descending aorta would receive an increased amount of mixed blood, with the arterial portion changed into venous and added to the venous portion as it entered the venous system to be carried to the right atrium.

There are two more diagrams here. D 20, which is a copy of D 14, shows the foetus before labour. The other, D 21, represents the foetus at the delivery, having lost the placenta, with the dilated right atrium and ventricle and venous congestion in the lower body.

Let us now consider the fundamentals of the second part. The foetus takes the first deep breath and the venous blood in the right atrium and the pulmonary

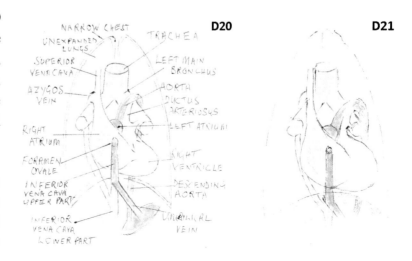

51

trunk is sucked up into the lungs, side by side with air entering the lung passages, leaving little venous blood for the lower body. But full expansion of the lungs could only occur if the blood entering the lungs is replaced by more venous blood from the lower body. So, by themselves, each part of the birth changes has a problem; in the first part the foetal lower body appears to have an excess of venous blood, and in the second part the lower body has too little. But put the two together and both problems are solved. I therefore now believe that the two parts of the birth changes are joined as one, and that as the foetus takes on blood from the placenta during the delivery, it takes the first deep breath at the same time, and as the venous blood from the right atrium enters the expanding lungs, it is replaced by the blood from the lower body.

But how will the foetus know when to begin breathing? This is difficult to answer. It must begin without delay after the delivery because the foetus has lost its blood supply, and it is usually accompanied with the arrival of consciousness, we must not forget that. I think there must be an inhibitory factor which prevents waking and breathing in utero, and after delivery it is cancelled and replaced by stimulation, which makes the foetus wake and breathe. Whatever the cause, breathing usually begins soon after delivery, and there must be a connection between those parts involved in respiration and waking, and those parts of the foetal brain which control breathing and consciousness.

The shock of entering the outside world would seem to be the cause of breathing, but could there be an intrinsic mechanism which stimulates the foetus to breathe after it has left the mother? My own ideas involve the dramatic diversion of the mixed blood from the placenta to the lower body at the delivery. Earlier, I have shown how the flow to the placenta would be larger than the flow to the lower body. The amount passing to the lower body would therefore be large, with the combined volumes of the right and left ventricles at 140 times each minute, or two and a half times each second, which is the usual foetal heart rate. The lower body includes many features; the lower spine, the abdominal and pelvic viscera, and the legs, with a large capacity widely distributed to receive the large amount transferred quickly.

I have found it difficult to accept that the respiratory centre in the brain stem could analyse the level of carbon-dioxide (CO_2) in the blood directly, because its blood supply would have been purified already by passage through the lungs, and it would be protected from the toxic effects of CO_2. I think there must be a sensory centre proximal to the lungs which can detect the level of CO_2 in the blood before it has passed through the lungs and relay the information to the respiratory centre, which could adjust the respiratory rate to an appropriate level. As I see it, the only appropriate place for the detection of the CO_2 levels would be the right atrium, where there is a confluence of all the venous blood arriving from the peripheral tissues. But the pacemaker controlling the cardiac output is in the right atrium. Is it possible therefore, for the right atrium to control not only the cardiac output, but the respiratory rate as well? (Here I am reminded that when I was a small boy, about seven or eight, I could slow my pulse rate by breathing out slowly. I cannot do it now because I have a pacemaker with a fixed heart rate). In which case any activity of the body would be matched by comparable increases in the heart and respiratory rates, under the eventual control of the cardiac and respiratory centres in the brain stem, and the large increase of venous return to the right atrium which occurs at the delivery would be detected in the atrium and stimulate the foetus to breathe, when it is outside the mother and safe to do so. Either way, the stimulation of the right atrium, or the shock of entering the outside world, would be followed by breathing. However, I strongly favour my own ideas, for a very good reason. The full inflation of the lungs requires a free flow of air into the respiratory passages, and a large amount of venous blood in the pulmonary arteries, the lungs cannot expand without both, and the large influx of venous blood into the right atrium would not only stimulate breathing but provide the right amount of blood for the lungs at the same time. *The cause of breathing, the eleventh hidden secret.* Earlier, I have described the delivery of the foetus and the taking of the first deep breath together as the 6th secret. But the delivery and the taking of the first deep breath are not hidden, we can all see them. It is the delivery of the *foetus* which is the 6th secret, and the taking of the first deep breath which causes all the changes when the baby is born, would be *the twelfth hidden secret.*

I have left the last paragraph intact without alteration because I have changed my mind. I now think there must be a common factor, and it would be the shock of leaving the comfort of the mother and entering the outside world which causes the breathing, and which would be *the eleventh secret.* In each case, a vaginal delivery and the Caesarean section, the foetus would breathe at the delivery, but with a vaginal delivery the mixed blood taken from the placental stream would have to pass through the tissues of the lower body, change into venous and enter the right atrium before allowing the lungs to expand fully, while the foetus plucked from the uterus may require some help with breathing before there is enough blood for full lung expansion.

Of course, the heart and lungs cannot work in isolation, they must be perfectly synchronised to bring energy to the body. The food is glucose, produced by the liver, and added to the right heart which pumps it to the lungs. In the respiratory capillaries, respiration occurs, CO_2 is given off and oxygen combines with the glucose to form liquid energy, and the left heart pumps it to every part of the body wherever it is needed. In the foetus it is different, the lungs are functionless, and the liquid energy, ready made in the placenta from the mother, is pumped by the left heart to wherever it is needed.

D22

It is important to understand that all the internal changes, circulatory and respiratory, take place quickly together. It may take me some minutes to describe the changes and take you more time to read and digest them, but as they all depend on the expansion of the chest and the descent of the diaphragm, *they must all take place at the same time,* as the first deep breath is taken by the foetus. They cannot be drawn out one after the other, though it may take more than one breath to inflate the lungs completely. Most important is the strong attachment of the inferior vena cava to the central tendon of the diaphragm, it is the place where circulatory and respiratory anatomy and physiology meet and ensures that the circulatory and respiratory changes are perfectly synchronised.

Let us consider the main features of the foetal circulation, illustrated in diagram D 22, which is a copy of D 14. The horizontal heart and the unexpanded lungs above the raised diaphragm. The narrow unexpanded cone shaped chest. The atria also raised above the diaphragm. The upper part of the inferior vena cava strongly fixed to the central tendon of the diaphragm above the liver and feeding the left atrium with arterial blood through the foramen ovale. The lower part of the inferior vena cava and the azygos vein feeding the right atrium with venous blood through the superior vena cava, and a block in the middle of the inferior vena cava. The ductus arteriosus meeting the aorta at the junction with venous blood, and the mixed blood in the descending aorta for the lower body and the placenta.

It is a pity that I have been unable to examine a foetal lamb this year, I had wanted to verify the relations of each of the foetal parts to one another, especially to confirm the position of the foramen ovale before and after birth, when it becomes the fossa ovalis. However, I have recently come across a collection of my drawings which I had made in May and

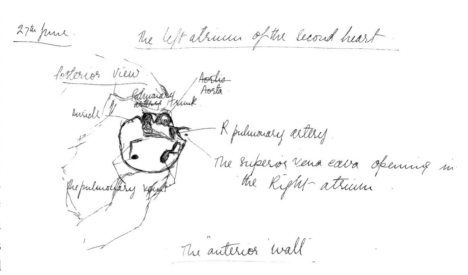

June 1968 in the anatomy room of our medical school, which more than compensates for a missing foetal lamb. I had tucked them away into a safe place before my move down to Horley last year. These drawings are very valuable and tell us about the foetal heart, the foramen ovale, and the blood flows through the heart. They were drawn in Indian ink, on the correct paper, and have been well preserved.

Let me show you the drawings of the left atrium.

The first shows the entrances of the four pulmonary veins outside the left atrium, while the other, below right which I have shown you before, shows the exits of the veins inside the atrium. The thin line drawn round the exits shows the limit of the atrium, and the two venae cavae would have been outside the atrium.

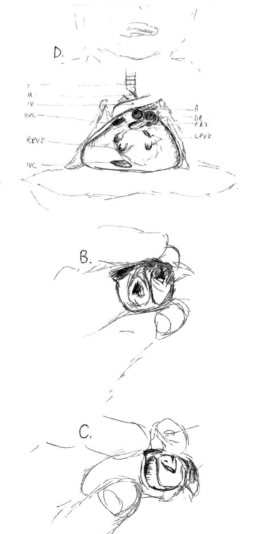

Drawing B shows the interior of the left atrium from above, with the atrioventricular opening on the left, and the septum primum of the foramen ovale on the right.

Drawing C gives a good view of septum primum on the medial wall of the left atrium, with the upper part of secundum beyond. The medial wall is also the interatrial wall, carrying the foramen ovale. To the left of the valve is the atrioventricular opening leading to the mitral valve and the left ventricle.

This drawing A, of the interior of the right atrium, is more interesting. It shows the inside of the atrium, with the foramen ovale on the medial wall of the atrium, which is also the interatrial wall. Clearly shown are the two parts of the valve, with septum primum surrounded by secundum. Below primum is a small mark I had made to show where the inferior vena cava would have been attached. To the left of the foramen ovale is a small face with a nose, and a mouth which is the opening of the coronary sinus draining the venous return from the heart into the right atrium. To the left of the nose is the atrioventricular opening

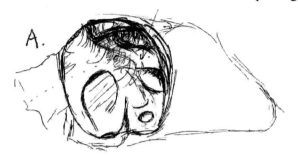

leading to the right ventricle, and further above is the opening of the auricle of the atrium. Before birth, the superior vena, attached to the upper right corner of this drawing, would be filling the atrium with the total venous return from the foetus, while the inferior vena cava would be passing through the venous blood, carrying the arterial blood to the foramen ovale and the left atrium.

We have now seen both sides of the foramen ovale. Septum primum separates the two atria, and a thin rim of secundum round primum completes the division between the atria.

If you will cast your mind back to picture P 29, you will see the remarkable connection between the coronary sinus and the unnamed branch of the inferior vena cava which feeds the lungs. They function as a pair, with a blade between them which acts as a valve, preventing backflow in atrial systole. Just as the leg muscles help to propel the venous blood back to the heart, the pulsating wall of the right atrium helps the coronary sinus to expel its venous blood into the right atrium in spurts, *it helps the circulation of the blood within the heart itself.* Likewise, the pulsating right atrium helps the inferior vena cava to expel its arterial blood in spurts through the unnamed branch into the right atrium, alongside the venous stream from the coronary sinus, and the combined stream flows into the right ventricle, one part to feed the lungs and the other to be replenished in the placenta.

We can now discuss the changes which occur during the transition from the foetus to a baby.

When the first deep breath is taken, the diaphragm moves down to a wider section of the cone, which becomes even wider with the expansion of the chest, with a sudden drop in pressure above the diaphragm and increased pressure below, which causes a rapid mass expansion of the lungs with air from the trachea, and venous blood from the right atrium, replaced by venous blood forced up from the lower body. The descent of the diaphragm pulls the inferior vena cava away from the foramen ovale, stopping the blood supply for the left atrium, which is quickly replaced by fresh blood coming from the lungs. The valve now separates the atria, each beating in time together without a flow between them, and the two septa become adherent, and are called the fossa ovalis. The reduced pressure above the diaphragm and the increased pressure below, forces the venous blood in the lower vena cava upwards as the upper inferior vena cava is pulled away from the foramen ovale, and the right atrium is filled with venous blood from both venae cavae. The diversion of venous blood to the lungs leaves none for the ductus arteriosus, which collapses and shrinks and changes into the ligamentum arteriosum, and none for the lower body which is then supplied with only arterial blood from the descending aorta, abolishing the segregation.

In diagram D 23 the foetus is taking the first deep breath. The opening lungs are being flooded with venous blood and air. The inferior vena cava is being pulled away from the foramen ovale, cutting off the arterial supply for the left atrium, and the lower venous return is being forced up into the right atrium behind the departing arterial blood for the left atrium. The ductus arteriosus is closing, stopping the venous blood supply for the lower body.

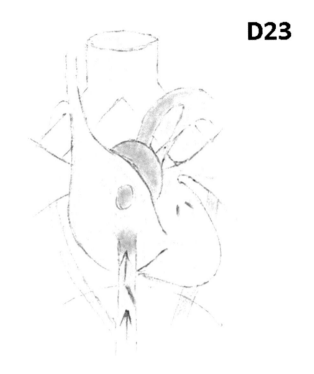

D23

Diagram D 24 shows the lungs filled with venous blood at the end of the first deep breath taken by the foetus when the baby is born, leaving none for the ductus arteriosus which closes, and none for the lower body which receives only arterial blood. Notice the elongated right atrium and the more vertical heart above the lowered diaphragm, the green ligamentum arteriosum, and the azygos vein which persists. Diagram D 25 shows the lungs bringing oxygenated blood to the left atrium during the next few heartbeats and the first deep expiration. Note the raised diaphragm, the more horizontal heart, and the tunnel valves in the left atrium.

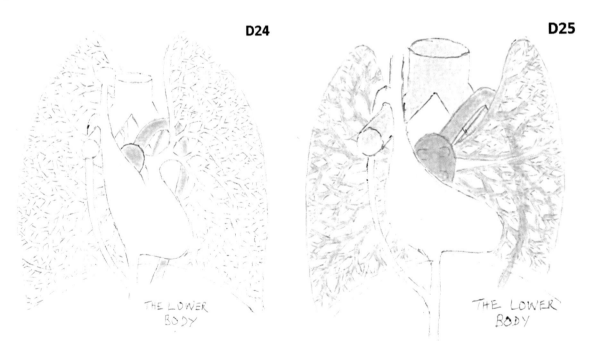

D24

D25

THE LOWER BODY

THE LOWER BODY

We will never again see such a deep breath; the diaphragm will remain in a lower position from where all future respiratory excursions will be made, but also, the diaphragm will have to descend from the raised foetal position, which will make the first deep breath even deeper.

The neonate continues to breathe, it has to, and the ductus arteriosus may take a few more days to close and become the ligamentum arteriosum, and the lower body becomes fully arterialised a little later to abolish segregation. There is more to come; the foetus has an easy time normally, being cared for by the heart, the placenta, and the mother, which allow it to respire without breathing. The heart rates of the boat race crews were 200 beats per minute, and the respiratory rates 40 per minute, giving a ratio of 5 to 1. In the older baby at rest, which we may call a postnate, the heart rate could be about 60 beats a minute, and the respiratory rate about 12 per minute, again giving a ratio of 5 to 1, and this ratio between the heart and respiratory rates would apply to a postnate of any age, with five heartbeats for each breath. And each beat of the heart would be accompanied by some of the aerated blood waiting to enter the pulsating left atrium through the tunnel valves, rather like the bag pipes, where there is always a reserve supply of air in the bag, waiting to enter the pipes.

In the foetus, without breathing, we cannot see a ratio between the foetal heart rate and respiratory rate, but there is a relation to the mother's heart rate, with the foetal heart rate of 140 being twice the mother's rate of 70 beats each minute, and each beat from the foetal heart for the foetus would be followed by another for the placenta.

During that first deep breath, the right heart will pump venous blood through the pulmonary arteries to the lungs five times, and five times will the pulmonary veins return arterial blood to the left atrium through the tunnel valves.

We can now list the precious secrets of the foetal circulation which have been revealed.

1. The inferior vena cava feeding the left atrium with arterial blood through the foramen ovale.
2. The ductus arteriosus leading to the side of the aorta with both vessels fusing together to form the beginning of the descending aorta.
3. The azygos vein, which persists after birth.
4. The division of the inferior vena cava into upper and lower parts.
5. The single superior vena cava feeding the right atrium with the total venous return.
6. The delivery of the foetus.
7. The segregation of the foetal circulation into two parts at the junction, with the upper feeding the upper body with arterial blood, and the lower feeding the lower body and placenta with mixed blood.
8. The unnamed branch of the inferior vena cava which feeds the foetal lungs with food and oxygen.
9. The tunnel valves of the left atrium, which persist after birth.
10. How the triple rhythm of the heart sounds in the foetus, indicates that the left atrium pumps blood into the left ventricle from the inferior vena cava.
11. The shock of leaving the comfort of the mother and entering the outside world, which causes the foetus to breathe.
12. The taking of the only first deep breath by the foetus, which causes all the changes as the baby is born.
13. The conversion of the foramen ovale into the fossa ovalis between the atria.
14. The change of the arterial blood supply for the left atrium, from the placenta to the lungs.

15. The filling of the right atrium with blood from both venae cavae, as the inferior vena cava is pulled away from the foramen ovale and leads venous blood from the lower body into the right atrium.
16. The elongation of the right atrium.
17. The diversion of the venous blood in the pulmonary trunk to the lungs, which changes the ductus arteriosus into the ligamentum arteriosum and removes the venous blood for the lower body, as segregation is demolished.
18. The blood supply for the placenta.

More thoughts on why the foetus breathes at birth.

During the five years I had spent in the rural districts of Africa and the four years in Fort Victoria, I had performed many Caesarean sections, it was the most common of my operations. I did not keep a record of the number I had done, but it would have been several hundred. However, throughout May 1967, I kept a record of the Caesars I had done in Fort Victoria, for a special reason. In 1954 when I was a house surgeon in Canterbury, the openings of the abdomens for the prostatectomies were not vertical, mid-line, but lateral, Pfannenstiel, suprapubic. It gave a better scar for the men. I decided to try it on the ladies for their Caesars. Also, I copied the Canterbury method of closing the skin with clips instead of sutures. I performed 27. If we call it 25, then the total for the year may have been about 300, and for my three years there without help, 900. If we add the many sections I had performed in the rural districts, the total may have been well over 1000. We did not have any serious problems making the 'babies' breathe, and they would have been cared for by the midwives. Nothing as bad as the little 'girl' who died in April 1965, most breathed spontaneously without assistance. So, why did they begin to breathe when I removed them from their mothers? And why were they able to breathe freely? The sectioned deliveries were quite different from the vaginal ones. I had said originally that the squashing of the placenta by the contracted uterus caused the mixed stream for the placenta to be diverted to the lower body of the foetus, and the resulting large venous stream for the right atrium not only caused the foetus to breathe but provided the right amount of blood for the lungs at the same time. But the sectioned 'babies' would not have had large venous streams for the right atria and would not have had the right amount of blood for the lungs to allow the lungs to open fully at the same time; or would they? I have to ask again, why did they breathe? Was it the removal of the warm amniotic fluid and the exposure to the outside air, or was it just that each foetus was able to recognise that it had left the mother and knew it had to breathe? Was it an inbuilt signalling mechanism which we all are provided with? As I have explained earlier, I now believe the reason why the foetus begins to breathe in both normal vaginal and sectioned deliveries is the shock of leaving the comfort of the mother and entering the outside world. But let me say more.

I have told you about the ruptured uteruses I had to deal with. In each case except one the foetus had died. Was it from lack of blood, or had it breathed and been asphyxiated by inhaled blood and amniotic fluid? Post-mortem examination of the lungs may have given us the answer, but at that time this problem had not entered my head. Let us look at that rare case where I was able to deliver a live baby because it had not breathed and been asphyxiated. Part of the placenta was still attached to the torn wall of the uterus and the foetus was receiving oxygen. We must not forget these facts, the connection with the uterus and the oxygen supply. The foetus would have escaped from inside the uterus to outside in blood and amniotic fluid, and the blood had not stimulated respiration.

I have introduced another plan of the circulation which separates the heart into two sides. They are normally joined as one because the right side must receive the arterial coronary supply from the left, the coronary sinus venous drainage of the left must empty into the right atrium, and they share the impulses from the pacemaker in the right atrium. Although the blood in the descending aorta is mixed homogeneous, I have separated it into arterial and venous to make things clearer. Earlier, I have divided the foetal changes into two parts, with the first part having an excess of venous blood in the lower body, and the second part having too little. But when they are joined together, they function as one, and when the foetus takes the first deep breath and the lungs

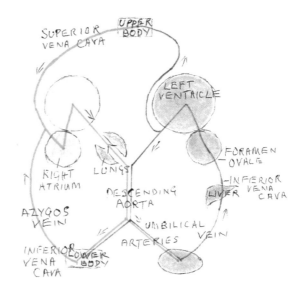

fill with air, they are also filled with venous blood from the right heart which is replaced by some of the venous blood from the lower body. *It is the venous blood in the lower body, which functions as a reserve throughout the later months of the gestation period, and which allows the sectioned 'babies' to breathe as well as the naturally delivered ones.*

Or is there something else to say? The little 'girl' who had died in Fort Victoria in April 1965, was of mixed African and another section of the human race. She passed into immortality anonymously as we worked to save her, and her body was taken to the mortuary where I was working on another body. Had I not been rewarded for performing the forensic work conscientiously myself, as her little heart began to uncover the precious secrets in a bedroom of my house? And had she not taken the last two secrets with her, of why she did not breathe at delivery, and why the foetus normally begins to breathe at birth?

Addendum. The steps taken as I assembled the path from the beginning to the end when the foetal circulation was finally uncovered.

Page 31. How I wondered in the mortuary, if the organs in a baby which had not breathed at birth, would be the same as those of a foetus. It led to my examination of the heart in my home, which showed it to be different from the orthodox view of two different streams of blood in the same chamber of the heart, and which showed the inferior vena cava leading arterial blood into the left atrium. This was the most important of my findings, which can be called the first secret to be uncovered. But if the inferior vena cava leads the placental stream into the left atrium, the venous return from the lower body must enter the right atrium by a different route.

Also on page 32, how I understood the importance of the ductus arteriosus, being as large as the aorta and gradually merging with the side of the aorta.

On page 35, the finding of the Azygos Vein was very important. It showed how the lower venous return could branch off the lower part of the inferior vena cava and enter the superior vena cava carrying the return from the upper body, and the superior vena cava would carry all the venous return from the whole body into the right atrium. The inferior vena cava must therefore be divided into two, the upper part to carry the arterial placental stream into the left atrium, and the lower part to carry the lower venous return into the right atrium, and there would have to be a block above the diversion to prevent the lower return from mixing with the left atrial flow. The azygos vein was the third secret, the block was the fourth, and the solitary superior vena cava carrying all the venous return into the right atrium, the fifth.

The next major revelation appears on page 39, where I reflect on the foetal features of the 'baby' who had died without breathing. Normally, the healthy baby would be delivered with the foetal features before breathing, then when the first deep breath is taken, all the foetal features disappear and are replaced by those of a live baby. The sixth secret would be the delivery of the foetus.

Further revelations follow quickly on the same page, when I had watched two television programmes. In the first, I had seen the delivery of a non-breathing animal which then had started to breathe, and I had seen a foetus change into a foal. In the second, I had seen the delivery of a goat kid, which remained without breathing. It was stillborn, and I had watched the delivery of a foetus. I then realised that stillborn farm animals could be a valuable source of information on the foetal circulation if human foetuses were unavailable.

On page 40, I describe for the first time, my findings in a stillborn lamb, and I was able to record them accurately with my first mobile phone. From my findings on the same page, I was able to make a plan of the foetal circulation. I followed this up by describing each section; the junction of the aorta and the ductus arteriosus, the circulations of the upper and lower bodies, and the circulation of the placenta. Finally, on pages 43 and 44, I was able to describe the blood supply for the foetal lungs and record it with my mobile phone.

My last contribution to this addendum appears on page 55, where I give my own account of the birth changes as I imagine them to be, when the first deep breath is taken by the foetus after delivery.